THE HEALTHY *Senior* WORKBOOK

This workbook contains personal health records and important medical information. If lost, please return to:

Name:_____

Address:_____

City_____State: _____Zip:_____

Telephone:_____

Barbara Lambesis
Editor

Marketing Methods Press
Phoenix, Arizona

Library of Congress Catalog Card Number: 91-061414

ISBN 0-9624798-1-0

Printed in the United States of America.

Preface

Good health is an essential ingredient in the recipe for a full and satisfying life. Poor health, due to illness or injury, quickly can rob seniors of their independence, dignity and even their purpose in life. Because we associate good health with access to medical care, everyone becomes concerned when the media warns of a crisis in the American healthcare system.

Politicians, insurance executives, medical professionals and healthcare administrators argue about the causes of and remedies for the problem of outrageously costly medical care. Yet, most overlook the need to involve the individual citizen, whose health is the topic of debate, as the key to the solution. Talking about instituting national health insurance or healthcare rationing makes headlines; encouraging people to take better care of themselves and to utilize medical services more effectively doesn't get votes or make news.

Actually, most illnesses and injuries requiring hospitalization and other expensive medical treatment to restore health can be avoided. Moreover, scientific studies taking place across the nation have demonstrated, without a doubt, that it is never too late for men and women in their later years to take steps to improve or maintain their health. So, if healthcare services are to remain affordable and accessible to all, everyone must assume greater responsibility for their own health. By adopting a healthy life-style and by improving communications with healthcare providers in an effort to get the best results from medical services received, individuals can live healthier lives and significantly eliminate much of the pressure on our costly and finite healthcare resources.

It's a simple idea, but a very powerful one. If individuals make commitments to take charge of their health, they can do more to maintain or improve their own well-being than all the healthcare debates and political posturing by Congress, all the complicated and costly health insurance plans in the marketplace and all the sophisticated medical technology currently available. Americans must stop expecting someone else to provide them with good health and must realize that following a healthy life-style and avoiding behavior patterns that can lead to illness and injury remain the responsibility of each person.

This workbook was compiled to help seniors stay vibrant, active and excited about their future. It provides age-specific health maintenance information and a method to monitor and manage health and medical records to effectively communicate with healthcare providers. It's a tool to help with the work of achieving good health in the years ahead...put it to good use and enjoy life!

Acknowledgements

Thanks to Ken Reinstein, Maribeth Brewer and Lori Yoney for their research and production assistance; to Dorie Roepke and the Auxiliary of Scottsdale Memorial Hospital for their consumer comments and insights that contributed to the development of this project; and to Ray Weinhold and Janet Runkle for their editing suggestions.

Gerald J. Jogerst, M.D., Oliver Harper, M.D., Marion Powell, R.N., M.C., Ann Hartwick, R.D., and Georgia Hall, M.P.H., Ph.D., reviewed the contents and made valuable suggestions that enhanced the text and strengthened the workbook's usefulness as a tool to improve communication between patients and healthcare providers. I'm grateful for their willingness to share their knowledge and expertise.

And finally, thanks to all the special seniors in my life, both friends and family. My wish for each of you to have a long, healthly and happy life was the inspiration for this book.

Barbara Lambesis
Editor

Table Of Contents

The information provided in this handbook is intended to complement, not replace, the medical advice given by your personal physician. For good health and safety, always carefully follow the advice given to you by your doctor and other healthcare professionals.

CHAPTER ONE

Taking Charge

A healthy lifestyle can prevent disease and injury throughout a person's entire life, and is especially important in later years. It is a misconception that there is little or nothing that can be done to preserve or protect good health in older adults. Scientific studies show that lifestyles and health habits at any age play important roles in maintaining good health and wellness.

So, no matter what your age, you can still take charge of your health. Do not be discouraged from doing the things that can help you feel better and maintain your health. It is never too late to accept responsibility for your well-being by adopting a healthier lifestyle and, as a result, getting more pleasure from life.

This handbook has been developed to help you maintain or even improve your health. It also provides easy methods for you to measure your progress.

Learn About Your Health

Take time to learn as much as you can about your health and about the normal aging process. By understanding the aging process, you will know what to expect and when to see a doctor about changes that may need attention. The information found in this handbook will describe many of the changes that occur during aging.

Physicians or other healthcare professionals with whom you feel comfortable and who can answer your questions are important sources of information. Two-way communication with your doctor is the best way to learn about your health. If you have a disease or illness, it is especially important to learn everything you can about it. Although not all diseases are curable, many can be treated successfully. Ask your doctor to explain carefully any tests or procedures being done. Have your doctor explain the purpose and side effects of prescribed medication and give details about any health problems you may have.

Many health organizations, such as the American Heart Association, American Cancer Society and the National Institutes of Health, also provide valuable information to the public about health problems. Many offer support groups, literature or educational programs.

Finally, learn what positive steps you can take to maintain or improve your health. Most steps are simple, common sense activities anyone can employ.

Develop A Healthy Lifestyle

No one needs reminding about how important health is to quality of life. Unfortunately, many people have surrendered responsibility for their health to doctors, hospitals, insurance companies and even the government. It's difficult, expensive and often painful to restore health once it is lost. Learning ways to avoid illness and injury and putting them to practice can help maintain or even improve a person's health. Since most illnesses and injuries are lifestyle related, making some simple changes can vastly improve a person's health and general well-being.

Part of a healthy lifestyle includes getting regular checkups. Screening examinations or tests should be done regularly for early detection of health problems. With early detection, many illnesses can be treated and cured effectively. Some tests may need to be performed more often, especially if you have an existing health problem or are at higher risk for developing certain diseases. Your doctor will be able to advise you about which tests are appropriate and how often they should be performed. Some tests may be done to provide a "baseline" record for future comparison. Later sections in this handbook provide general information about routine tests and a place to keep health records.

Keep Good Records

Don't rely on your memory alone to keep track of all the information that relates to your health. Utilize the designated pages in this book for documenting this information. Information recorded should include: health professionals you have seen and why; illnesses or surgeries; medications you are taking; allergies; special diets or treatments you require; the dates of your immunizations or examinations; your height, weight, blood pressure; and progress toward achieving a healthier lifestyle. There are special sections throughout this handbook in which to keep this information.

Because healthcare is costly, know what kind of coverage your health insurance plan(s) offer. If you need tests or surgery, check your plan's requirements. These might include the need to get a second opinion or to check with the insurance provider before going to the hospital. Also, keep selected insurance information in this handbook for easy reference. Review your insurance plan(s) often to make sure your coverage is adequate and current.

Common Theories On Aging

Scientists are seeking knowledge about how the human body ages constantly, but exactly how and why aging occurs still remains a mystery. Most scientists believe that aging is a complex process involving many body systems. Through their research, they hope to discover what can be done to slow the process. Scientists have developed several theories in pursuit of answers to the questions of human aging.

Most theories on how aging occurs focus on what happens in the body's cells as time passes. All cells change over time and as a result lose their ability to function. Aging occurs as more and more cells are altered or changed. One theory of aging suggests that cell changes are due to genetics - cell attributes inherited at birth. Changes in cells that lead to maturity, aging and death follow a set, predetermined timetable, according to this theory.

Another theory indicates that aging is caused by damage occurring to cells in various body systems throughout life. Such damage could be caused by "wear and tear," harmful substances that we breathe and eat, or natural processes within the body. The "damage" theory holds promise that cell changes might someday be corrected or avoided and life expectancies extended if appropriate preventive measures are taken.

A third theory suggests that aging results from slowly occurring damage to the DNA in body cells. DNA directs the machinery of every cell. Eventually, DNA damage would cause cells, then body tissues and organs, to break down or die.

Changes in body hormones are responsible for aging, according to another theory. At some point, a gland such as the pituitary, releases a hormone (or fails to produce one) and aging begins, according to this theory.

The immune system is the focus of yet another theory. The immune system is the body's weapon for fighting disease. As people grow older, this system becomes less effective, opening the way for infection by viruses, bacteria, and other disease-producing organisms. As the immune system ages, it also tends to lose the ability to differentiate between the body's own tissues and foreign substances. As a result, cells of the immune system that once would fight invading organisms now attack the body itself, producing diseases.

While scientists continue to explore how and why the human body ages, it is unlikely they will find a practical way in the near future to extend life or prevent aging completely. So, it's important to adopt a sensible approach to protecting your health and dealing with aging.

Leading A Healthy Lifestyle

There are no known "anti-aging" treatments, drugs, or supplements that slow down the aging process or extend life. You can improve your chances of staying healthy and living longer if you:

Get Regular Exercise
Stop Smoking
Wear Your Seat Belt
Eat Right
Prevent Injuries
Protect Against The Sun
Avoid Infection
Limit Alcohol Consumption
Watch Your Weight
Control Stress
Get Enough Rest
Be Positive/Enjoy Others

The Fountain Of Youth Does Not Exist

Over the years, many people have been swindled purchasing magic potions, special devices or other products to restore youth or prevent aging. Check with a doctor before buying a supplement or making a dietary change. Be suspicious of any product that promises to slow aging, extend life or produce major changes in appearance or vigor. To date, there is no scientific evidence that supports most claims for "Fountain of Youth" remedies.

Aging - The Normal Process

As you grow older, your body and mind will undergo a number of physical and mental changes. The changes you experience may be perfectly normal or they may signal health problems that you should report to your doctor. You should not expect unusual aches or pains or melancholy just because you are older. Unfortunately, many seniors think aging means health problems and accept a decline in health when, in fact, most problems are due more to a lack of exercise, not eating the right foods, smoking or to treatable illnesses than to aging.

So, What's Normal?

Everyone will experience some physical and mental changes as they grow older. But, normal changes that occur do not necessarily cause illness, disease or disability. Some of the things people can expect as they grow older are:

Changes in Sight

Farsightedness is normal as eye muscles weaken with age and the elasticity of the lens decreases. In addition, the lens of the eye often yellows, and the pupils do not let in as much light. More light may be needed to read and reading glasses may be necessary.

Changes in Skin

The number of sweat glands decreases with age, leading to drier skin. The skin also becomes less elastic and has less supporting tissue causing wrinkles. Deep wrinkles and very dry skin are more common among those who have overexposed their skin to the damaging rays of the sun.

Decrease in Bladder Capacity

When a person grows older, the kidneys do not filter blood as efficiently and bladder capacity decreases. Loss of urine, discomfort when urinating or other symptoms are not necessarily normal and should be reported to your doctor.

Minor Aches and Pains

Joints that have been used extensively over a lifetime may experience a loss of cartilage. For some, this may lead to mild arthritis or occasional aches or pains in the joints. These discomforts usually can be remedied with non-prescription pain relievers. Severe pain or stiffness, however, is not normal, and you should contact your doctor if you experience these symptoms.

Changes in Sleep Patterns

It is a myth that older adults need more sleep. Seniors do experience less dreaming than younger adults and may wake up more often during the night or awaken earlier in the morning. Nevertheless, healthy older adults do not require greater amounts of sleep. The amount of sleep required for good health should remain relatively constant through adulthood.

Hair Loss and Graying

Some thinning of the hair is normal. In addition, most hair becomes gray as a person grows older. The extent of the hair loss and the onset of graying are usually determined by hereditary factors.

Changes in Hearing

While some loss of hearing high-pitched sounds is normal, severe hearing loss is not and you should consult a physician if you experience this problem. Often, some or all of the hearing loss can be restored with proper diagnosis and treatment.

Changes in Taste

Aging causes a decrease in the number of taste buds and a reduction in the amount of saliva produced. As a result, older adults may notice a decrease in the ability to taste some food flavors and may need to increase seasonings to enjoy the taste of food.

Hardening of the Arteries

As you age, arteries usually become less elastic and the inner lining of the artery can thicken. The thickening is caused by an accumulation of fatty substances on the inside wall of the arteries. When this occurs, blood flow can be restricted, causing a slight rise in blood pressure.

Changes in Stature

Many people lose one or two inches in height as they age. This is due to a gradual loss of bony tissue in the spine, a condition that is more prevalent among women. Any loss in height greater than one or two inches is not normal and is a reason to consult your doctor.

Slight Changes in Mind Power

While older adults have a slightly slower reaction time and may take longer to absorb and understand new material or concepts, retention of new information should be equal to that of younger people. Some forgetfulness is normal at any age, but any significant change in mental function is reason to consult a doctor.

People who remain healthy in their later years can enjoy more independent, fulfilled lives. To help your doctors and other health professions evaluate your ability to function adequately, complete the "Health Check - - Activities of Daily Living" chart on the following page.

Complete the "Health Check" every six months and be sure to report any changes in your activity level to your physician.

Health Check--Activities of Daily Living

Score yourself every six months on the activities of daily living listed below. Place a "Y" for Yes and "N" for No in the appropriate box.

Are you presently able to:

DATE:

1. Get to places out of walking distance?				
2. Handle shopping needs?				
3. Do daily housework?				
4. Prepare and cook full meals?				
5. Handle daily finances?				
6. Get out of a chair without assistance?				
7. Walk without a cane or walker?				
8. Walk without the fear of falling?				
9. Dress yourself?				
10. Groom yourself adequately?				
11. Control bladder and bowel functions?				
12. Bathe yourself independently?				
13. Regulate your own medications?				
14. Live in an independent setting, such as your own house or apartment?				

CHAPTER TWO

GET REGULAR EXERCISE

Exercise Is For Everyone

Exercise isn't just for athletes or young people! It's for everyone who wants to improve or maintain health. A beneficial exercise program does not require special equipment, a health club, or class participation. All you need is the will to get started and a sensible program. Regular exercise is essential if you want to take good care of yourself.

No Age Barriers

Recent studies show that with exercise even the very elderly and frail can realize significant improvement in strength and mobility. Whatever your age, you'll see and feel the improvement exercise makes in your health and general well-being.

Get Started With A Simple Program

It's easier to get started and stay with an exercise program if it's kept simple and involves an activity you enjoy. Try to make exercise a regular part of each day. Set goals and use the exercise diary at the end of this chapter, noting each day you exercised, what activity was done, for how long and your pulse rate. Reward yourself at regular intervals for following your routine and reaching your goals: rent a favorite movie, enjoy a play or buy that new piece of clothing you've been admiring as a reward for sticking to your program.

Safety First

Be sure to consult your doctor before starting an exercise program, especially if you have heart or other health problems! Always remember-- safety first. Forget the slogan "no pain, no gain." Pain associated with exercise is usually an indication that something is wrong. If pain is experienced, slow down or stop completely. While exercise can be beneficial to people of any age, certain medical conditions may limit the amount or type of activity appropriate for each individual. Using the wrong kinds of exercise may cause injury or be dangerous. Start exercising slowly. Later, when you know your limits, do more. Dress according to climate conditions for comfort and protection, keeping in mind that very hot or very cold weather can strain your system.

Everyone Needs Exercise For:

A Healthy Heart. Regular exercise strengthens the heart. A fit heart reduces the risk of heart disease and stroke. In addition, a fit heart doesn't have to work as hard to deliver the amount of oxygen needed by the muscles during activity.

Weight Control. Exercise is ideal for weight control. It burns calories, which in turn can take off pounds so a desirable weight can be maintained.

Energy. Exercise increases energy levels, helping you get more out of life.

Better Sleep. Exercise reduces tension, promotes relaxation and helps promote a more sound, restful sleep.

Muscle Tone. Different types of exercise help shape and tone specific muscle groups for a slimmer, trimmer you! Muscles that are exercised are more efficient.

Walking--A Great Way To Start

Walking is an exercise almost everyone can do and is one of the best ways to start an exercise program. It's easy and, best of all, it's effective. Brisk walking gives the heart an excellent workout, and a good pair of walking shoes is the only equipment needed. Walking is a pleasant activity that can be done alone or with others. If you are a beginner, start with a moderate walking program, then move on to other, more vigorous exercise activities once you build strength and endurance.

A good walking program requires proper walking techniques. To achieve the full benefits of walking, posture should be upright and arms should swing rhythmically. The stride should be comfortably long, using the hip and leg muscles to "push" your body along.

Set a brisk pace. Try walking with a friend and observing each other's walking style. Practice good techniques to become a more efficient walker and help each other to improve.

Good shoes are essential for comfort when walking. Look for a shoe that is wide enough to fit the ball of your foot with plenty of room for your toes to move. Many companies manufacture shoes that are specially made for walking and are stylish, too. Well-cushioned soles are important since they serve as shock absorbers. Laced shoes adjust easily for comfort and fit. Thick, absorbent socks (preferably cotton) complete the walker's footwear. Don't forget to bring your walking socks with you when buying walking shoes!

Walking also gets you out of the house and into fresh air and sunshine. Even urban dwellers can enjoy observing signs of nature on a daily walk. While gaining the benefits of exercise, one can observe seasonal changes in the landscape and may encounter such wildlife as birds and squirrels. Walking can be a pleasurable experience, as well as a healthy activity for the body.

Once you have mastered a brisk walk, try jogging, swimming, bicycling, dancing or low-impact aerobic calisthenics if your doctor concurs. These activities can deliver healthful benefits, as well as a sense of accomplishment and well-being.

Exercise To Stay Fit

To gain maximum health benefits, exercise must be done regularly, but not overdone. Follow the "FIT" formula developed by the National Heart, Lung, and Blood Institute.

"F" stands for **FREQUENCY**, or how often you exercise. For the heart and lungs to benefit from exercise, working out three to five times each week is recommended.

"I" stands for **INTENSITY**, or how hard you work during the routine. A workout should challenge you, but not exhaust or push you to your limit. Try the talk test. If you can hold a conversation while exercising, you're doing great. If not, slow down. Also, check your heart rate frequently to gauge exercise intensity. You must achieve your target heart rate during exercise to receive the full benefits. Heart rate target zones are listed later in this chapter.

"T" stands for **TIME**. To exercise the heart, each workout should last at least 20 minutes. A beginner may start with a 10-15 minute session and gradually work up to 20-30 minutes.

Check Your Heart Rate

It is important to keep track of your heart rate during exercise. Your heart will beat faster when exercising than when at rest. How fast it should beat during exercise depends on your age, exercise intensity and fitness. Everyone has a recommended heart rate target zone. The number of heartbeats per minute reached while exercising should fall within your target zone to make exercise worthwhile and safe.

It's important to reach and maintain your target zone to achieve a healthier heart. However, working out above your target zone is too hard on your heart. Find your target zone in the following table by looking for the age closest to yours and reading across the line.

Heart Rate Target Zones

AGE (Years)	TARGET ZONE (Beats Per Minute)
50	102-145
55	99-140
60	96-136
65	93-132
70	90-127
75	87-123
80	84-119
85	81-115
90	78-111

To find the exact target zone for your age use this equation. Subtract your age from 220, then multiply that number by 60% and by 85% to find the bottom and top of your target heart rate. Your doctor may suggest a heart rate target zone different from the beats per minute listed on the above chart. Be sure to get your doctor's advice before starting your exercise program.

When working out, allow time for your heart and breathing rates to rise gradually. Then check your pulse regularly during the routine to see if you've reached your target zone. If you don't know how to check your pulse, ask at your doctor's office and a health professional will show you.

Take Some Precautions

Some cautions are worth mentioning. An increased breathing rate is to be expected when exercising, but if you experience the following symptoms:

Extreme shortness of breath
Chest pain
Dizziness
Nausea
Profuse sweating with extreme fatigue

slow down or stop to make sure your body returns to normal quickly. In addition, if you experience any of these symptoms, report them to your physician before resuming the same level of activity.

You may experience some muscular soreness for a few days after beginning a new activity. But if you have:

Severe pain that doesn't go away
Joint swelling
Limited joint motion

your body may be telling you to slow down and let the healing process take over. You may resume the activity when the condition improves if your doctor approves.

To avoid injury, start any new exercise slowly and increase gradually. It's worth repeating: "Listen to your body and act accordingly." Exercise should make you feel better, not worse!

The Challenge

Regular exercise is one of the best ways to take good care of yourself. The hardest part of exercising is getting started and sticking to it long enough to realize the benefits. The person who has been sedentary for many years will find it takes several weeks to realize the benefits of exercise and the sense of well-being and enjoyment it can bring. In the beginning, it may just seem like hard work. The rewards, however, are certainly worth the effort.

So, start feeling good and looking better, with a sensible, regular exercise program. Use the charts that follow to measure your progress and help you set and reach your exercise goals.

Exercise Log

DAYS		1	2	3	4	5	6	7	TOTALS	COMMENTS
Sample	Activity	Walk		Walk		Walk	Walk		Walk	Enjoyed walking in the morning with my neighbor. Saw a robin.
	Distance	1 mi.		1 mi.		1.5 mi.	1 mi.		4.5 mi.	
	Time	18 min.		17 min.		26 min.	17 min.		78 min.	
	Heart Rate	105		106		110	108		107 Avg.	
WEEK 1	Activity									
	Distance									
	Time									
	Heart Rate									
WEEK 2	Activity									
	Distance									
	Time									
	Heart Rate									
WEEK 3	Activity									
	Distance									
	Time									
	Heart Rate									

Exercise Log

WEEK	DAYS	1	2	3	4	5	6	7	TOTALS	COMMENTS
WEEK 4	Activity									
	Distance									
	Time									
	Heart Rate									
WEEK 5	Activity									
	Distance									
	Time									
	Heart Rate									
WEEK 6	Activity									
	Distance									
	Time									
	Heart Rate									
WEEK 7	Activity									
	Distance									
	Time									
	Heart Rate									

Exercise Log

DAYS		1	2	3	4	5	6	7	TOTALS	COMMENTS
WEEK 8	Activity									
	Distance									
	Time									
	Heart Rate									
WEEK 9	Activity									
	Distance									
	Time									
	Heart Rate									
WEEK 10	Activity									
	Distance									
	Time									
	Heart Rate									
WEEK 11	Activity									
	Distance									
	Time									
	Heart Rate									

Exercise Log

	DAYS	1	2	3	4	5	6	7	TOTALS	COMMENTS
WEEK 12	Activity									
	Distance									
	Time									
	Heart Rate									
WEEK 13	Activity									
	Distance									
	Time									
	Heart Rate									
WEEK 14	Activity									
	Distance									
	Time									
	Heart Rate									
WEEK 15	Activity									
	Distance									
	Time									
	Heart Rate									

Exercise Log

DAYS		1	2	3	4	5	6	7	TOTALS	COMMENTS
WEEK 16	Activity									
	Distance									
	Time									
	Heart Rate									
WEEK 17	Activity									
	Distance									
	Time									
	Heart Rate									
WEEK 18	Activity									
	Distance									
	Time									
	Heart Rate									
WEEK 19	Activity									
	Distance									
	Time									
	Heart Rate									

Exercise Log

WEEK	DAYS	1	2	3	4	5	6	7	TOTALS	COMMENTS
WEEK 20	Activity									
	Distance									
	Time									
	Heart Rate									
WEEK 21	Activity									
	Distance									
	Time									
	Heart Rate									
WEEK 22	Activity									
	Distance									
	Time									
	Heart Rate									
WEEK 23	Activity									
	Distance									
	Time									
	Heart Rate									

Exercise Log

DAYS		1	2	3	4	5	6	7	TOTALS	COMMENTS
WEEK 24	Activity									
	Distance									
	Time									
	Heart Rate									
WEEK 25	Activity									
	Distance									
	Time									
	Heart Rate									
WEEK 26	Activity									
	Distance									
	Time									
	Heart Rate									
WEEK 27	Activity									
	Distance									
	Time									
	Heart Rate									

Exercise Log

DAYS	1	2	3	4	5	6	7	TOTALS	COMMENTS
WEEK 28 Activity									
Distance									
Time									
Heart Rate									
WEEK 29 Activity									
Distance									
Time									
Heart Rate									
WEEK 30 Activity									
Distance									
Time									
Heart Rate									
WEEK 31 Activity									
Distance									
Time									
Heart Rate									

Exercise Log

DAYS			1	2	3	4	5	6	7	TOTALS	COMMENTS
WEEK 32	Activity										
	Distance										
	Time										
	Heart Rate										
WEEK 33	Activity										
	Distance										
	Time										
	Heart Rate										
WEEK 34	Activity										
	Distance										
	Time										
	Heart Rate										
WEEK 35	Activity										
	Distance										
	Time										
	Heart Rate										

Exercise Log

	DAYS	1	2	3	4	5	6	7	TOTALS	COMMENTS
WEEK 36	Activity									
	Distance									
	Time									
	Heart Rate									
WEEK 37	Activity									
	Distance									
	Time									
	Heart Rate									
WEEK 38	Activity									
	Distance									
	Time									
	Heart Rate									
WEEK 39	Activity									
	Distance									
	Time									
	Heart Rate									

Exercise Log

DAYS		1	2	3	4	5	6	7	TOTALS	COMMENTS
WEEK 40	Activity									
	Distance									
	Time									
	Heart Rate									
WEEK 41	Activity									
	Distance									
	Time									
	Heart Rate									
WEEK 42	Activity									
	Distance									
	Time									
	Heart Rate									
WEEK 43	Activity									
	Distance									
	Time									
	Heart Rate									

Exercise Log

DAYS	1	2	3	4	5	6	7	TOTALS	COMMENTS
WEEK 44 Activity									
Distance									
Time									
Heart Rate									
WEEK 45 Activity									
Distance									
Time									
Heart Rate									
WEEK 46 Activity									
Distance									
Time									
Heart Rate									
WEEK 47 Activity									
Distance									
Time									
Heart Rate									

Exercise Log

DAYS		1	2	3	4	5	6	7	TOTALS	COMMENTS
WEEK 48	Activity									
	Distance									
	Time									
	Heart Rate									
WEEK 49	Activity									
	Distance									
	Time									
	Heart Rate									
WEEK 50	Activity									
	Distance									
	Time									
	Heart Rate									
WEEK 51	Activity									
	Distance									
	Time									
	Heart Rate									

CHAPTER THREE

Stop Smoking

There is irrefutable proof that smoking contributes to heart disease, emphysema and cancer and is a major cause of premature, preventable death in the United States. An estimated 85 percent of lung cancer cases in men and 75 percent of the cases in women are caused by cigarette smoking. And, according to a recent Surgeon General's report, smoking is responsible for one out of every six deaths in this country.

If you are one of the 13 million American smokers over 50, it's time to quit! Even if you have been smoking for many years, you still can benefit from quitting and reverse some of the ill effects of the habit.

Louis Sullivan, U.S. Secretary of Health and Human services, said in 1990, "Even if one has smoked for nearly half a century, stopping now will add years to your life, as well as life to your years. Your body can repair much of the damage smoking has done, if you stop."

"Within one year after quitting, the extra risk of dying from a heart attack caused by smoking is gone," Sullivan said. "Within months of being smoke-free, the heart and circulation begin to improve."

There are other benefits you can realize from quitting. Sleeping patterns will improve, contributing to a more sound, restful sleep. Breathing capacity should improve and you should be able to walk longer without shortness of breath. People with smoking-related conditions, such as emphysema and chronic bronchitis, may see their conditions stabilize once they quit. Finally, quitting will save you money -- money that you will be able to enjoy -- smoke free.

Smoking Shortens Your Life

According to the Surgeon General's Report, "Reducing the Health Consequences of Smoking, 25 Years of Progress," smoking claims 390,000 lives every year and is responsible for one out of every six American deaths. Recent studies show that smoking will reduce the average life span of a male by one-fourth. A male smoker dies at the average age of 64, instead of 82.

Smoking Increases Your Risk Of Cancer

It is a fact that smoking causes cancer. Lung cancer was the first form of cancer to be directly linked to cigarette smoke. The chances of getting lung cancer increase every time a person lights up. Other factors that increase the risk of cancer among cigarette smokers include the number of cigarettes smoked daily and the tar and nicotine content of cigarettes smoked. Research also has linked smoking to cancer in several other areas of the body including the mouth, esophagus, bladder, kidney, stomach, cervix and pancreas.

Smoking Damages Your Heart And Lungs

Smoking definitely contributes to emphysema, heart disease and other circulatory ailments. Nicotine in cigarettes causes a narrowing of the arteries that reduces circulation everywhere in the body. Years of smoking damages the heart muscle and increases the risk of a heart attack. Moreover, smoking is the leading cause of emphysema, a lung disease that slowly destroys breathing capacity. Emphysema damages lung tissue and progressively destroys the respiratory system. People with emphysema may spend years gasping for air or clinging to an oxygen tank.

Quitting Isn't Easy

If you have tried to quit smoking, but started again, you are not alone. Most ex-smokers tried at least three times before successfully breaking the habit. The best way to approach a renewed attempt at quitting is to use your past failures as a learning experience. Examine what went wrong, draw on the experience, set a date to quit and make the attempt again.

Here's some interesting information about the myths associated with breaking the smoking habit.

In the past, it was believed that people who quit on their own, without support groups or formal programs, were more successful at remaining smoke-free. However, new data shows little difference between those who quit solo and those who seek support to break the habit.

Some doctors also have prescribed drugs for those addicted to cigarettes. However, when various drugs used to combat nicotine withdrawal symptoms were studied for their effectiveness, scientists found that the only effective treatment for nicotine withdrawal was the use of nicotine itself in the form of chewing gum. The gum requires a prescription, and becomes habit forming. However, when combined with a stop-smoking program, the gum has been shown to be somewhat successful at getting people to quit inhaling cigarette smoke.

Whether you are trying to quit for the first time or the fifth time, here are some tips from the National Heart, Lung, and Blood Institute that can help you take care of yourself and those around you, too, by giving up smoking. Getting started is the hardest part.

Tips To Help You Stop Smoking

1. Write down all the reasons you should stop smoking. Post that list in a conspicuous place, where you will see it. Read the list whenever you have an urge to light up.

2. The next time you want to smoke, wait 15 minutes before lighting up. Then try waiting 20 minutes, then 30 minutes and longer when you feel the urge to smoke.

3. Set a specific date for quitting completely. Tell everyone about it, so they can support you. Your friends, family and co-workers can be a great support group for your effort.

4. Throw out all your cigarettes, lighters, matches and ashtrays to keep you from giving in to temptation. Whenever you get the urge to light up, eat a carrot or other low-calorie snack that will keep your mouth busy. Try taking a walk, chewing sugarless gum, eating some fruit or drinking some cold water whenever you crave a cigarette.

5. Find something to keep your hands occupied. Write or type a letter, play with a coin or paper clip, twirl a pen, buy a yo-yo, add up the money you are saving from not smoking on a calculator. Exercise, talk to a supportive friend or take a deep smoke-free breath to take your mind off the urge to smoke.

6. Once you have survived the withdrawal symptoms, you'll need to adjust your entire lifestyle to stay off nicotine. Plan new activities, different forms of relaxation, and try changing eating and exercise habits to keep from gaining weight. You also may have to avoid

temporarily friends who smoke, to keep yourself from wanting to light up.

7. Reward yourself for goals reached. Try to go a certain number of days without smoking and then do something special for yourself. Buy a piece of clothing, attend a concert or treat yourself to something special as a reward for your efforts. Quitting isn't easy, it takes hard work and mental toughness. When you make progress, you should reward yourself.

8. You also might want to take a stop smoking class to help you break your smoking habit.

What If You Cheat?

It takes time to break a habit, especially one as addictive as smoking. If you have smoked for the majority of your life, quitting won't be easy.

If you do light up, don't give up your effort because you smoked one cigarette. Regain control of yourself and analyze what led you to smoke again. Then establish a contingency plan, in case you find yourself reaching for a cigarette. Live and learn from the experience. Think of all the advantages to being smoke-free and renew your commitment.

Use the chart on the following page to list your reasons for quitting, the date you intend to quit completely and the things you will do if you get the urge to smoke.

Reasons I Should Quit Smoking:

_____

_____

_____

_____

_____

_____

_____

_____

Date I'm Going To Quit:

_____

When I Have The Urge To Light Up, I'm Going To:

_____

_____

_____

_____

_____

CHAPTER FOUR

Eat Right

Good nutrition is an important part of taking good care of yourself. This is especially true as you get older. Eating the proper amount of fiber, limiting saturated fats and foods high in sodium and cholesterol, and getting enough of the appropriate nutrients are important activities for maintaining proper weight and for preventing high blood pressure, blocked arteries, heart attacks, strokes, malnutrition and some types of cancers.

Many of the health problems people face as they get older have been linked directly and indirectly to the types and amounts of foods they eat. For example, obesity is associated with high blood pressure, high blood cholesterol, diabetes, heart disease and stroke. In addition, one-third of all cancer deaths may be related to our diets, according to the National Cancer Institute.

Six different nutrients essential to healthy living are found in various foods. The United States Recommended Daily Allowance

(US RDA) is the standard by which consumers can determine if they are getting enough of these nutrients from the foods they eat daily. The following is an explanation of each nutrient and its benefit to your health:

Proteins -- Proteins are the body's building blocks. They are essential for growth, replacement and maintenance of cells and they form the hormones and enzymes that regulate the body's processes. Extra protein not used by the body is transformed into body fat or used as an energy calorie supply. According to the US RDA, a male adult over 50 years of age requires 63 grams of protein each day and a female adult of the same age requires 50 grams daily.

Carbohydrates -- This nutrient includes dietary fiber, starches and sugars. Dietary fiber is responsible for regular waste elimination, and starches and sugars are the main energy suppliers for the body. It is recommended that 50-60 percent of food an adult eats each day should be from the carbohydrate group.

Fats -- Fats also are energy suppliers, as well as transporters of fat-soluble vitamins. Some fats, in addition, also help form cell membranes and hormones. They are the most concentrated source of calories, therefore, fat intake should be limited to no more than 30 percent of the daily total caloric intake.

Vitamins -- The body needs these organic substances in very small amounts. Vitamins are not energy suppliers. However, they act as a catalyst for the release of energy from carbohydrates, fats and proteins, as well as acting as catalysts for other internal chemical reactions.

Minerals -- Minerals build strong bones and teeth, produce hemoglobin in red blood cells and maintain body fluids. Like vitamins, these nutrients aid in internal chemical reactions and are needed only in small amounts. They do not supply energy. Adults should attempt to eat foods that will supply the recommended daily allowances of vitamins and minerals and avoid relying on supplements.

Water -- Yes, water is a nutrient, too. It serves as the transportation system for the other five nutrients, regulates body temperature and helps remove waste. Water also replaces body fluids lost in urine and sweat. Doctors encourage adults to drink at least eight, 8-oz. glasses of water each day.

Many of the foods we eat contain various ingredients that affect our health. Depending on the ingredient, we should either increase or cut back our daily intake to stay healthy and prevent disease and illness. The following ingredients have been found to impact health.

Sodium

There is an established link between our intake of sodium and high blood pressure. Salt is the main source of sodium in the diet, but not the only one. Sodium can be found in many foods, especially processed foods and dairy products, where it is used to flavor and preserve. Some sodium is beneficial to the diet, helping to maintain normal blood pressure and blood volume by bringing water into the blood vessels. The recommended daily intake of sodium is only 1 to 3.3 grams, or 1/2 to 1- 1/2 teaspoons of salt. This amount is well below the daily intake of the average American.

There are many ways to reduce your daily sodium intake. Try cutting back on the condiments and salt-seasonings you add to foods. Condiments and seasonings such as ketchup and mustard; steak, soy, Worcestershire and barbecue sauces; garlic, celery and onion salt; baking powder and soda; and salad dressings are high in sodium. Avoid frozen dinners, dehydrated soups and sauces, canned soups and any processed foods to lower your sodium intake. Reduced sodium versions of these products may be used moderately.

Beware of foods that claim to be "low- or no-salt." They may contain other forms of sodium which you also should avoid. Learning to read product labels is important if you want to cut back on sodium and other food ingredients such as cholesterol and saturated fats.

Cholesterol And Saturated Fats

Cholesterol and saturated fats are two ingredients that should be reduced or eliminated from your diet. These ingredients are found primarily in such animal products as meats, poultry, butter, lard and animal shortening. Certain vegetable oils also are high in saturated fats. Avoid coconut, palm and cocoa oils, as well as cocoa butter.

High levels of blood cholesterol and saturated fats have been linked to the development of high blood pressure and arteriosclerosis, a narrowing of the arteries causing reduced blood circulation. A reduced flow of blood can lead to a stroke or heart attack.

The amount of cholesterol in the bloodstream, including that which we get from the foods we eat and that produced naturally by the body, should not be above a count of 200, or 200 milligrams (mg) of cholesterol per deciliter (dl) of blood. This is the "count" that is often talked about when cholesterol levels are checked by your doctor or at health clinics and health fairs held in local communities.

It is important to get your cholesterol level checked regularly. Keep records of your cholesterol count in the medical records section at the end of this book. If it is high, you may bring it down by changing your eating habits to avoid fats and saturated fats, as well as foods that are naturally high in cholesterol. Having a high level of blood cholesterol increases your risk of heart disease. For example, someone with a blood cholesterol level of 265 mg/dl has a four times greater risk of heart disease than the person who has a level of 190 mg/dl.

Limiting foods high in cholesterol and saturated fats can be one of the important things you can do to maintain a healthy heart and circulatory system.

Fiber And Starch

Fiber and starch are important parts of your diet. You may remember your mother telling you to eat plenty of roughage when you were younger. Your mother knew what she was talking about. She was simply telling you to eat enough fiber, which is the part of plant foods that your body cannot digest. The average person's daily intake of fiber is about 11-12 grams, which is not enough according to the National Cancer Institute. The recommended diet includes between 20-30 grams of fiber each day.

There are many benefits to eating enough fiber. Fiber acts as a laxative, helping to move waste products through the body quickly, relieving constipation and possibly diluting certain cancer promoters, such as high-fat foods, thus protecting the colon from cancer. It also may be beneficial in the prevention of diabetes, heart disease and obesity. The validity of these benefits, however, is still being studied.

Starch, or complex carbohydrates, is a fine source of dietary fiber and essential nutrients. Foods high in starch may be much lower in calories than foods composed of simple carbohydrates or sugars and contain little or no nutritional value.

Good sources of fiber and starch include whole grain breads and breakfast cereals, whole-wheat pastas, potatoes, corn, white rice, brown rice, dried beans, peas, lima beans, fruits and vegetables with edible skins, stems and seeds.

There are several different types of fiber. Eating a variety of foods containing fiber, such as cellulose, pectin, lignin and gums, is important to make sure you are getting the health benefits of all the various fiber types.

Sugar

While diabetes, obesity, acne and even heart disease have been blamed on sugar, scientific studies show no direct link to anything but tooth decay. Sugar, however, is high in calories and has little nutritional value. People who eat diets high in sugar often are not receiving enough of the other nutrients necessary for good health which are provided in a balanced diet.

Sugar is not just the white refined type commonly found on the table. All forms of sweeteners containing calories are considered sugar. Other forms include brown sugar, raw sugar, corn syrup, honey and molasses. Additionally, other forms of sugars such as corn-based sweeteners and sucrose also are added to foods during processing.

Read the labels of the foods you buy to avoid too much sugar in your diet. Avoid foods containing corn syrup and high-fructose corn syrup, honey, lactose, mannitol, molasses, maple syrup, maltose, glucose, fructose, dextrose and, of course, sugar. Instead choose natural sources of sugars in fruits, vegetables, milk products and some cereals.

Obtain Vitamins From A Balanced Diet

Some studies have shown a connection between diets rich in vitamins A, C and beta-carotene (a natural form of vitamin A found in plants) and a lower risk of getting certain cancers. The National Cancer Institute recommends a diet that includes foods rich in these nutrients, and cautions people not to rely on vitamin supplements entirely.

Dark green vegetables are a good source of vitamins A and C. Try eating broccoli, spinach, endive, kale, chicory collard greens, beet greens, turnip greens, mustard greens, chard, dandelion greens and watercress. Also, vitamin A can be found in deep-yellow vegetables such as carrots, pumpkin, sweet potatoes and winter squash. These vegetables also are good sources of beta-carotene.

Eat A Wide Variety Of Foods

What you eat is an important part of staying healthy, especially as you get older. It is extremely important to eat balanced meals, including a wide variety of foods from the four food groups. Eating meals that are nutritionally balanced, low in fats, sugar and sodium and high in fiber and complex carbohydrates can help you improve and maintain your health.

The Four Food Groups

Milk Group -- Includes milk, cheeses, yogurt, ice cream and ice milk. Adults should have a minimum of four servings daily. Select low-fat milk products.

Meat Group -- Includes lean meats, fish, poultry, eggs, dried peas, dried beans, nuts and seeds. A minimum of two servings daily is recommended.

Fruit-Vegetable Group -- Includes fruits and all varieties of vegetables. Adults should eat at least four servings daily.

Grain Group -- Includes breads, pastas, rice and grains. A minimum of four servings daily is recommended.

Poor Eating Habits

The results of a 1990 survey indicate one in five elderly Americans often skip one or more meals daily and that 33 percent of those surveyed said they did not care about eating a proper diet. The survey results, released by the Nutrition Screening Initiative, also mentioned that 45 percent of those surveyed take multiple prescription drugs. These drugs could affect a person's appetite, ability to taste and/or the nutritional benefits of foods eaten.

If you fit the description of the people surveyed in this poll, it is time to change your eating habits. If you do not already eat properly, or often skip meals, you might see a significant improvement in the way you feel, your energy level and your health in general if you start eating properly.

Reading The Product Label

If you are on a restrictive or weight loss diet, or if you are just concerned about the foods you eat, always read the nutrition information on the package when selecting foods. Even so, that information can be misleading or hard to understand because of the difference between such terms as "light" and "lean" or "sell date" and "expiration date." Only foods that make a nutrition claim or have vitamins, minerals or nutrients added are required to have a nutrition label, and only about half the foods in the supermarket are labeled.

It is important to understand fully what all the information means. For example, a food that claims to have no salt may contain one or more of 70 different sodium compounds used in the processing of foods.

Also, labels refer to food only as it is packed, which sometimes differs from how it is eaten. If you have to add something to the food before you cook it, the nutritional composition changes.

CHAPTER FIVE

Watch Your Weight

Maintaining ideal weight is important at any age. There are many health benefits to keeping your body fit and trim. Staying trim reduces the risks of heart disease, cancer, high blood pressure, diabetes and other medical problems associated with being overweight. You can increase your chances of living longer and having more energy for desired activities if you control your weight. Moreover, you'll probably be more happy with your appearance if you don't put on unnecessary extra pounds.

The following weight tables give ranges for men and women according to height. Please note the tables list average weight ranges. Your weight may not be in the ideal range due to your activity level, build, health and physical condition. If you are outside the ideal range for your height and sex, it does not mean necessarily that your health is in jeopardy. Consult your physician for a personal analysis of the ideal weight range for you. To use the weight tables, find your height and determine which column lists your weight.

If your weight falls at or below the number in Column A, it is in the ideal range. A weight in column B is considered 1-19% over the ideal range, and a weight in column C is 20-39% over the ideal. Weight in column D is more than 40% over the ideal range.

Your goal should be to achieve and maintain ideal weight. If your weight is in column B, C, or D, ask your doctor whether you should begin a weight reduction and control program.

If your weight is not within the ideal range listed for your height, your doctor may suggest a change in your diet and an exercise regimen depending on whether you need to lose or gain weight to reach your ideal range.

Ideal Height/Weight Range Based on Metropolitan Life Tables

Height	A Ideal	B 1-19% Over	C 20-39% Over	D 40% Over
WOMEN				
4'7"	Less Than 94	94-112	113-131	132 & Over
4'8"	97	97-115	116-135	136
4'9"	100	100-119	120-139	140
4'10"	103	103-123	124-143	144
4'11"	106	106-126	127-147	148
5'0"	109	109-130	131-152	153
5'1"	112	112-132	133-156	157
5'2"	116	116-137	138-161	162
5'3"	120	120-142	143-167	168
5'4"	124	124-147	148-173	174
5'5"	128	128-152	153-178	179
5'6"	132	132-156	157-184	185
5'7"	136	136-161	162-189	190
5'8"	140	140-166	167-195	196
5'9"	144	144-171	172-201	202
5'10"	148	148-176	177-206	207
MEN				
5'0"	Less Than 116	116-137	138-161	162 & Over
5'1"	119	119-142	143-166	167
5'2"	122	122-145	146-170	171
5'3"	125	125-149	150-174	175
5'4"	128	128-153	154-178	179
5'5"	131	131-156	157-182	183
5'6"	135	135-161	162-188	189
5'7"	140	140-167	168-195	196
5'8"	144	144-172	173-201	202
5'9"	148	148-177	178-206	207
5'10"	152	152-181	182-212	213
5'11"	157	157-187	188-219	220
6'0"	161	161-192	193-224	225
6'1"	166	166-198	199-231	232
6'2"	170	170-203	204-237	238
6'3"	175	175-209	210-244	245
6'4"	180	180-215	216-251	252

Losing Those Extra Pounds

Promotions and advertisements for weight loss clinics, diet plans, diet drinks and diet pills are everywhere in the marketplace. Before-and-after pictures of people who have lost 100 pounds or more are blazoned, larger than life, on outdoor billboards in major cities. These advertisements attempt to lure new customers with touching testimonials about the effectiveness of each diet plan.

Because every weight loss program being advertised and promoted has its own convincing success stories, Americans spend millions of dollars every year on plans and programs promising fast results. Some plans can cost hundreds of dollars and may work only temporarily. Often the lost weight is gained back several weeks or months later, leaving the dieter as heavy or heavier than before. If you need to lose weight, it is important to choose a diet plan that will be safe and effective.

With so many different diet plans available, choosing the best and safest option can be confusing. If you are overweight and want to lose those extra pounds, be very cautious. No matter what diet program or plan you choose, be sure to pick one that will help you lose weight without jeopardizing your health. Check with your doctor to make sure you pick a safe and effective plan.

Cutting Calories

Calories are a count of the energy received from the food you eat. Your body uses calories as an energy source to perform its routine daily functions, as well as fight off disease, regulate body temperature and repair injuries. To perform these functions, an average 51- to 75-year-old man needs approximately 2,400 calories per day while the average woman in the same age group needs approximately 1,800 calories.

Beware of any diet that limits you to an intake of less than 1,000 daily calories, unless it is medically supervised. To safely lose weight, the average person should reduce their caloric intake by approximately 500 calories per day. By doing so, 3,500 unused calories, or one pound of weight, will be cut from a person's diet over a seven-day period.

When you diet, it is important to eat right. To maintain a healthy body, you should eat foods from each of the four food groups to make sure you get all the nutrients required to properly maintain your body.

The four food groups are:

1. Meat and Poultry
2. Milk and Dairy Products
3. Breads and Grains
4. Fruits and Vegetables

Some of the "quick" or "gimmick" diets on the market today restrict the intake of certain food groups, which may cause a person to be tired or weak. To maintain your health when dieting, limit calorie intake, not the intake of foods from each of the four food groups.

You can lose weight effectively by eating a variety of foods from all the groups. However, your choice of food is the important concern. Each group has foods that are highly nutritional, yet low in calories. Careful selection of foods, smaller portions and proper food preparation are the principles of successful weight loss.

Avoid foods with high fat content. Try eating less fried foods since frying foods in fats and oils adds considerable calories. Instead, try broiling or baking foods and trim away excess fat and skin from meats before cooking. Removing the skin or breading from fried foods makes little difference in reducing the fat or calorie content, since the food absorbed the extra fat during the frying process. Also, try drinking skim or 1% milk instead of other types of milk with higher fat content.

Take Off Extra Pounds Slowly

It is recommended that you lose no more than one or two pounds per week. If you eliminate 3,500 calories per week from your diet by eating foods that are low in calories and high in nutrition, you can shed one pound each week.

One pound a week does not seem like much, when there are diets that promise a loss of "20 pounds in 20 days." However, most of the weight lost during the first few weeks of dieting is water weight, which is the easiest to lose and the fastest to gain. Also, if you attempt to lose weight too fast, your body may think it is starving and take up the defensive, trying any way it can to signal you to eat. Once you give in to your body's request for food, you often gain back more weight than you had originally lost. This type of weight loss has been labeled "yo-yo" dieting, and is now being called a major eating disorder. Remember, the slower you lose weight, the better chance you have of keeping it off.

Tips For Losing Weight

The best method for successful, healthy weight loss does not involve diet pills or rigid food plans, just some very simple advice.

1. Start by keeping records of your food intake. Measure all portions and keep track of the exact amount of food you eat. This may seem cumbersome, but many people do not have a clear idea of just how much they actually eat until they start measuring and recording. Use the chart at the end of this chapter to help you record all the foods you eat for one week.

2. Try drinking a glass of water before meals. This will make your stomach feel fuller, leaving less room for other foods.

3. Don't bring serving bowls or plates of food to the table. This might tempt you to take that extra serving you don't need.

4. Eat slowly. Your brain takes 15-20 minutes to realize that something is in your stomach. If you are having problems slowing down your eating habits, try using your opposite hand or try eating with a pair of chopsticks.

5. You can eat many of the same foods that you have always eaten, just eat less. Try different methods of food preparation and exercise more to help you lose weight and firm up.

6. Weigh yourself only once a week at the same time of the day and be consistent about eating or not eating before you get on the scale. This will give you a more accurate picture of your weight since it fluctuates depending on the time of day, what you have eaten that day and whether or not you have exercised. Keep a record of your weight loss and reward yourself for pounds lost.

Eating Little And Often vs. Three Square Meals A Day

There are conflicting views on whether it is better to eat three times a day or to eat six or more small meals daily. Research from early studies suggested that a decrease in body fat corresponded with an increase in the number of small meals eaten. The scientists involved found that successful weight loss resulted from eating less total food with several mini-meals than with three big-meals.

In other studies where calorie intake was equal between those eating six or more meals and those eating three times a day, results showed that mini-meal eaters lost more weight and/or body fat.

A 1987 study by the United States Department of Agriculture Western Human Nutrition Center in San Francisco found different results. Regardless of whether participants consumed three large meals or six or more smaller meals, their bodies burned calories at the same rate.

Research on this subject is difficult to carry out due to the number of variables involved. The amount and type of food eaten, the subject's activity level, body metabolism, and the degree of a person's obesity all make conclusive research difficult.

Dieting by eating six or more mini-meals is not recommended for people who are considered obese, since it is harder to track food intake and the method may promote constant eating. Remember when trying to lose weight, it's not how or when you eat calories, but the amount consumed and the amount burned during exercise or other activity that accounts for weight gain or loss. You may wish to experiment with each approach to determine which works better for you and makes you feel better.

Common Activities That Burn Calories

Exercising is important for maintaining your health and your ideal weight. The more you exercise, the more calories you burn and the more pounds you can lose. The following chart shows the approximate number of calories burned during some very common activities based on the approximate energy expenditure of a healthy adult male weighing 150 pounds.

Activity	Calories per hour	Activity	Calories per hour
Aerobic Dancing	600	Rollerskating	300
Bicycling	240-420	Sitting quietly	95
Calisthenics	360	Skiing - cross country	600
Canoeing	360	Skiing - downhill	500
Dancing	240-420	Sleeping	55
Golf	250	Swimming	540-660
Horseback riding-trot	350	Table tennis	170
Housework	190	Tennis - singles	420
Ice skating	300	Walking	240-450
Jogging	480		
Officework	140		

Values on the preceding chart are approximate. Individual results may vary depending on weight, physical condition, age, gender and activity level. Ask your physician if you have any questions about exercise and its impact on your weight control program.

Use the following charts to record your food intake, monitor your weight and adjust your activity to use up calories and lose weight.

Food Intake Diary

Record the types and amounts of foods you eat and the total calories consumed each day. Keep records for one week to determine your eating habits before you start a diet.

	Breakfast	Lunch	Dinner	Snacks	Total Calories
Day 1					
Day 2					
Day 3					
Day 4					
Day 5					
Day 6					
Day 7					

Weekly Weight Record

Weigh yourself once a week at the same time of day to get the most accurate picture of your weight.

Date\Time	Weight		Date\Time	Weight

Weekly Weight Record

Weigh yourself once a week at the same time of day to get the most accurate picture of your weight.

Date\Time	Weight

Date\Time	Weight

CHAPTER SIX

Avoid Infection

People battle bacterial and viral infections throughout their lives, combating common infections with bed rest, fluids, pain relievers and antibiotics. For the most part, infectious diseases such as colds and flu are of little concern. That's because after a few days of suffering from minor aches and pains, sneezing, a runny nose or a slight fever, health usually returns without complications. As a person ages, however, infectious diseases pose a greater health threat and precautions should be taken to avoid them.

A common infection that may have simply kept you home from school for a few days in your youth may be a serious concern as you become older. Infections, such as influenza and pneumonia, can lead to serious health complications if not properly taken care of by a doctor or healthcare professional. Furthermore, if someone is already suffering from a serious or chronic illness, common infectious diseases can lead to serious complications and become life-threatening.

No one is completely immune to infectious diseases. We are constantly assaulted by airborne, waterborne and foodborne bacteria and viruses. The severity of infections contracted by coming in contact with infectious organisms can range from mild to life-threatening, depending on an individual's physical condition, general health, immune system, and extent of the contact with the organism.

The body has many defenses to fight off infection and illness. Externally, body oil, perspiration, tears, saliva and mucus are the first line of defense. Coughing and sneezing are other ways the body fights organisms attempting to penetrate body tissues and cause infection. If organisms get past the front lines, components of our skin, saliva, cells, circulatory system and blood provide another level of defense against infection and illness.

If a virus or bacteria survives the first two lines of defense, the body puts its immune system into action. The immune system is made up of lymph nodes, the spleen, areas of the gastrointestinal tract and bone marrow. While the first two defense mechanisms attack infectious organisms in general, the immune system concentrates on the specific type of invading organism, utilizing defenses designed to counterattack a single type of infection.

Common infections that can be especially dangerous to older adults are influenza and pneumonia.

Influenza

Each winter, millions of people suffer from the unpleasant effects of influenza, commonly known as the "flu." The normal treatment for this viral infection affecting the nose, throat and lungs is a few days of rest, over-the-counter pain relievers and plenty of fluids. For the healthy person, the flu is usually a mild disease. But for older people, or someone with a chronic illness, the flu can be life-threatening by lowering one's resistance to other more serious infections, such as pneumonia.

The flu is passed easily from person to person when someone sneezes or coughs, sending droplets containing the virus into the air to be picked up by others through their respiratory system. Flu symptoms include weakness, headache, backache, cough and fever, lasting one to six days. The appearance and severity of the symptoms vary from one person to another. Some people experience no symptoms at all, while others may suffer from chills, sore throat, aching muscles and red, watery eyes.

These symptoms are very similar to those associated with the common cold, also caused by a virus. Colds are generally shorter in duration than the flu and are not accompanied by a fever.

Influenza is rarely a fatal illness. However, secondary infections such as pneumonia brought on by the flu can be life-threatening. Older people, especially those already suffering from heart disease, emphysema, asthma, bronchitis, kidney disease or diabetes, are most at risk for developing a secondary infection. As a result of the debilitating effects of another illness, the immune system may not be strong enough to resist a secondary infection while fighting the flu.

Treatment of the flu is related to whatever symptoms are present. Usually your doctor will recommend aspirin or a similar pain reliever for aches and pains, bed rest until the fever is gone, and plenty of fluids to prevent dehydration. A persistent fever or cough could indicate a more serious condition. If they occur, you should contact your doctor to prevent the development of further complications.

Preventing The Flu

The U.S. Public Health Service recommends a yearly immunization to combat various flu strains that appear each season. In order to build up sufficient immunity, it is best to get immunized in early November, before the start of flu season. In addition, it's best to avoid other people who are suffering from the flu until they have fully recovered.

Pneumonia

Pneumonia is one of the most common secondary infections associated with the flu. It can be life-threatening and is one of the five leading causes of death among people over the age of 65. Pneumonia is an inflammatory condition of the lungs which can be caused by a flu virus or, more often, by bacteria that has multiplied while the body was fighting a flu infection.

Pneumonia's symptoms are similar to those associated with the flu, but are more severe. Coughing is more frequent and may produce a colored discharge. Shaking and chills can be common, and a severe fever, remaining from the flu infection, may continue. Pain in the chest can occur, along with a shortness of breath, due to inflammation of the lungs.

A doctor should be contacted promptly if an individual is experiencing persistent fever or other symptoms associated with pneumonia. Antibiotics can be an effective treatment for pneumonia, if taken early in the course of the disease.

Prevention of some types of pneumonia is possible with an immunization against pneumococcal diseases. This is a one-time vaccine recommended by the U.S. Public Health Service for the elderly or those with chronic illness. A low fever and local soreness are occassional side effects of the vaccine, but are minor and short-lasting. This immunization can be given at the same time as the flu vaccine without additional side effects occurring.

Bronchitis

Another less dangerous secondary infection associated with the flu is acute bronchitis. Bronchitis, an inflammation of the bronchial tubes, also can appear on its own and is most prevalent in the winter. Bronchitis can be caused by both viral and bacterial sources and can be serious to a person already suffering from a chronic disease. Also, if someone already has lung, coughing or bronchial problems, respiratory failure may result from the onset of bronchitis.

Symptoms include fever, sore throat, chest pain and a cough. Treatment may include medications such as cough medicine, antibiotics, an increase in fluids, rest and the use of a humidifier for steam.

Preventing Infection

Many infections can be prevented by taking some simple precautions.

Practice Good Hygiene

It never hurts to be reminded about the importance of practicing some very basic, good hygiene habits. Keeping yourself clean by washing and bathing regularly, brushing your teeth and changing and cleaning your clothes often can help reduce your chances of contracting infectious diseases. Always wash your hands with warm water and soap after using the toilet and before preparing and eating food. Always cover your nose and mouth when you sneeze or cough and carefully dispose of tissue you have used to blow your nose to prevent spreading disease.

Eat Right

Proper nutrition is important for resisting infection, too. If you eat a well balanced diet, your body will have more energy to resist the bacteria and viruses that cause infection. Fueling your body with nutritious foods will reduce your chances of becoming ill and may shorten the recovery time if you do get sick.

Food Preparation

To avoid having disease-producing bacteria multiply in food, follow a simple rule. Always keep hot foods hot, and cold foods cold. Do not allow foods to stand at room temperature for long periods and keep all foods covered both in and out of the refrigerator or freezer. Storing foods properly and keeping cooking utensils and work areas clean also can reduce chances of food contamination.

Get Enough Rest

Getting enough rest also is important for staying healthy. Most people need seven or eight hours of sleep each night to be fully rested and to fight off organisms that cause infectious diseases.

Avoid Close Contact With Sick People

If possible, avoid people who are sick with colds, flu or other infectious diseases. By doing so, you will reduce your chances of becoming ill. Talk to an ill person by telephone, rather than visiting in person. Don't get close to someone who is coughing or sneezing. Don't share food, drinking glasses or utensils with a sick person. Caregivers should take extra precautions when caring for people with infectious diseases.

Keep Immunizations Current

Check with your doctor to make sure your immunizations are current. While flu and pneumonia shots are very important, your doctor may recommend that you be protected against diphtheria, whooping cough, tetanus and polio, as well.

CHAPTER SEVEN

Preventing Injuries

The United States leads the world in trauma-related deaths, according to the National Safety Council. Almost 150,000 people lose their lives annually as a result of accidental injuries. These injuries contribute to the high cost of medical care in America, accounting for more than $150 billion in medical expenses, lost income and productivity each year.

As people age, their coordination, balance, muscle strength, vision and hearing may change or diminish. These reduced capabilities can make older adults more prone to accidental injuries that can result in permanent disability or even death.

Many injuries common to older adults can be prevented by taking simple precautions. Avoid driving at night and always wear a seatbelt when riding in a vehicle. Make sure your home is safe and free of hazards that could lead to a fall or other serious accident. Be aware of the side effects of the medications you take. Many prescription drugs, or combinations of drugs can cause drowsiness and slower reflexes making an older adult more vulnerable to accidents.

Drive Safely, Wear A Seat Belt

According to the National Highway Transportation Safety Administration, if you live to 75 years of age, your chances of being involved in an auto accident resulting in injury during your lifetime are greater than 86 percent. If you are involved in a motor vehicle accident, wearing a seatbelt can save your life and prevent or reduce the severity of injury. More than two-thirds of the states in the U.S. currently require seatbelt use for front seat occupants. Seatbelt use has been credited with saving an estimated 12,000 lives annually.

You should always wear a seatbelt, no matter how short a time you plan to be in the car. A majority of serious auto accidents involving injury happen within 25 miles of the driver's home, at traveling speeds of less than 40 miles per hour. Passengers not wearing seatbelts have a three times greater risk of injury requiring hospitalization and are two-and-a-half times more likely to have serious injuries requiring medical transportation to a hospital than those who buckle up.

Don't Drink And Drive

In addition to wearing a seatbelt, do not drink and drive. More than half of all fatal traffic accidents studied involved alcohol. A driver impaired by alcohol is significantly more likely to be involved in an accident.

Make Recreation Safe

Older adults usually have more time for recreational activities than their younger counterparts, so receational safety becomes an important concern. All recreational activities require the use of common sense and safety practices to prevent injuries. For example, when involved in any water-related activity such as canoeing, boating, fishing and rafting, always wear a life preserver or carry a personal flotation device, especially if you cannot swim. Drinking alcohol while driving a boat or recreating on the water is just as dangerous as drinking while driving an auto!

Bicycling is another activity that older adults enjoy. However, most people fail to consider the potential danger of bicycle riding. Every year bicyclists suffer an estimated 70,000 serious head injuries. These injuries can be avoided by wearing a bicycle helmet. You are twice as likely to require hospitalization if you ride a bicycle without a helmet and are involved in an accident. Helmets cost between $39-60, are light-weight and comfortable and should be worn whenever bicycling. There are different types of helmets made for different riding surfaces and styles. Ask for help at a bicycle store to get the right helmet for your riding needs.

Home Safety Tips

Safety precautions in your home are essential. You can eliminate many potential injury-causing hazards in your home with a routine safety check. For example, a loose throw rug, rickety chair, dark hallway or slippery shower are hazards that can be easily eliminated to make your home safer.

Home safety is especially important for older women who are prone to osteoporosis, a bone thinning disease which makes bones brittle and susceptible to breakage. Many falls, and their associated injuries, can be prevented by making a few simple changes around the home, and taking a few sensible safety precautions.

Here are some tips to make your home a safer place to live and to reduce the chances of accidental injury.

The Kitchen

In the kitchen, make sure all regularly used cupboard items are at or below eye level and within easy reach. Repair or replace all frayed or cracked appliance cords to prevent electric shock and keep all appliances properly maintained. Also, put large handles on doors, utensils and cookware for easier grasping.

The Living Room

In the living room or den, repair rickety chairs and furniture, cover sharp corners and make sure that all furniture is stable and easy to get in and out of. If needed, install handrails along the wall or keep a cane or walking device nearby to reduce the possibility of a fall. Always keep walkways free from such obstructions as magazines, newspapers, shoes and other items. If you have large sliding glass doors or big picture windows, put decorative decals or stickers on them to help you determine if they are open or closed.

The Bedroom

In the bedroom, avoid sleeping in high beds. If you have a motorized bed, always keep it in the low position. Make sure you have a lamp and a telephone with a lighted dial within easy reach of the bed to avoid having to search for them in the dark. Finally, if you smoke, remove ashtrays from the bedroom to avoid the temptation to smoke in bed where you could fall asleep and start a fire.

The Bathroom

The bathroom has many potential hazards. If needed, install an elevated toilet seat and put handrails on the walls by the toilet. Handrails also are important in the bathtub or shower. Make sure that you use non-slip mats or decorative appliques in the tub or shower stall to prevent slipping. Use non-skid rugs to avoid walking on wet, slippery surfaces in the bathroom.

Besides making each room in your home hazard free, there are many other precautions that will help make your home as safe as possible.

Good lighting in all parts of the living quarters is essential. Make sure that light switches are easy to reach at the bottom and top of stairs, next to the bed, in the bathroom, kitchen, den and garage. Make sure there is always enough light for you to see where you are going and detect anything in your way. Many accidents can be avoided by installing brighter light bulbs or adding more light fixtures in your home.

Sturdy handrails also are important to install up and down the length of stairways. Make sure they are securely fastened at the proper height to give maximum support.

Keep common living areas free of such hazards as electrical cords, low tables, grandchildren's toys, glasses or newspapers, which might cause you to fall or trip. Also, make sure that rugs are secure and chairs are heavy and stable enough to support your weight.

Balance And Coordination

Good health and regular exercise can help maintain or improve your balance and coordination, thus helping to prevent accidents. Exercise can help you maintain muscle tone, strengthen bones and keep joints, tendons and ligaments as flexible as possible. Being agile helps prevent dangerous falls and may reduce the severity of injuries if you are involved in an accident.

Vision and hearing can affect balance and coordination, too. Have both checked regularly and, if necessary, remedy any discovered problems or conditions. Sometimes, problems with balance may be helped by simply removing a buildup of wax from the ears.

Prescription and non-prescription drugs also can affect

coordination and balance. Ask your doctor or pharmacist about the drugs you are taking and any possible side effects, especially if you are taking more than one type of medication.

Alcohol definitely affects motor skills and can further aggravate existing balance and/or coordination problems. Never consume alcoholic beverages before you drive an auto or operate any machinery or appliances.

Climate control in your home is important to your health and safety, too. If a home is too cold, the low temperature can cause a person to feel dizzy and disoriented, leading to falls. For comfort and safety, your home's temperature should not fall below 65 degrees Fahrenheit.

What you wear on your feet also can affect your balance. Wear supportive, rubber soled shoes, with low heels. Avoid walking in socks or smooth-soled shoes, especially on slippery or waxed floors.

A cane, walker or walking stick can help you maintain footing if you have problems with your balance. Use special caution when you are not familiar with your surroundings, or if outdoor surfaces are wet, icy or uneven.

In summary, many dangerous falls and accidental injuries suffered at home or while recreating can be avoided by removing home hazards and taking sound safety precautions.

SAFETY QUIZ

Answer the questions "Yes" or "No" to determine if your home is safe and if you are using routine safety precautions in your daily living. Consider making some adjustments to your home if you cannot answer "Yes" to each question.

1. Do you have the local emergency phone number 911 for ambulance, fire and police available by your telephone? _____

2. Are your telephones about waist high for an easy reach? _____

3. Do you have handrails by each set of stairs? _____

4. Do you have a smoke alarm in your home? _____

5. Do you use a rubber mat or appliques in your bathtub or shower? _____

6. Are your throw rugs fixed to the floor by tape or Velcro? _____

7. Are the floor surfaces level between rooms in your home? _____

8. Do you have adequate lighting in every room of your home? _____

9. Is there a light within easy reach of your bed? _____

10. Are items you routinely use stored on shelves within easy reach? _____

11. Are your home's most traveled areas free from small pieces of furniture or other floor obstructions? _____

12. Do you have decorations clearly marking glass doors? _____

13. Do you have a telephone within reach of your bed? _____

14. Is there a handrail on the wall by the toilet and/or bathtub? _____

15. Do you know the side effects of the medication you take? _____

16. Do you always wear your seatbelt when riding in a car? _____

17. Do you always use a life preserver or flotation device when recreating on the water? _____

18. Do you avoid swimming or exercising alone? _____

19. Do you always wear a helmet when riding a bicycle? _____

20. Have you avoided a falling incident in the past six months? _____

CHAPTER EIGHT

Get Enough Rest

Sleep recharges your body, giving you the energy needed to function from day to day. The amount of sleep required should remain relatively consistent throughout adulthood. Nevertheless, 40 percent of Americans over the age of 60 have problems getting enough rest -- either waking up throughout the night or not being able to go to sleep. Some suffer from a sleep disorder, but most simply have poor sleeping habits.

Sleep problems are not due to aging alone. According to a study by the National Institute of Health, disease, emotional distress and poor sleeping habits are the leading causes of sleeplessness among the elderly.

Many turn to medications to solve the problem. Experts caution that over-the-counter sleep medications often are ineffective and can be counter-productive. The drugs may make the user feel sleepy, but they often have adverse side effects and don't treat the basic cause of sleeplessness. Prescription drugs, likewise, may not be appropriate in many cases of sleeplessness.

If dramatic changes in sleeping habits occur, it is wise to consult your doctor. There are many side effects associated with not getting enough sleep. Falling asleep at the wheel of a car is a leading cause of automobile accidents on the nation's highways, second only to alcohol. Lack of sleep also can lead to dangerous mistakes, even when doing the most common and routine activities. In addition, people who are not well rested often are irritable and unpleasant.

Most people require about seven to eight hours of sleep per night, although amounts vary widely depending on individual needs. Sleep consists of two different cycles: Rapid Eye Movement (REM) and non-REM. During REM sleep, which is very light, dreams occur. The deeper sleep cycle, non-REM, does not include dreaming, and as you get older, the amount of time spent in this stage decreases. This explains why older adults are considered light sleepers.

If you are not getting enough rest at night, you may just need to change your daily routine. Or, you may be suffering from a sleep disorder.

Sleep disorders affect up to 50 million Americans. Insomnia is the most common complaint, affecting people at any age. If it takes more than 30 minutes to fall asleep, or if you wake up often and can't go back to sleep, you may have insomnia. Most of the time, insomnia is a symptom of stress or anxiety, and not a physical problem.

Sleep apnea is another common sleep disorder which affects breathing. A person with apnea may stop breathing for up to two minutes, several times nightly, without realizing it. There are two types of apnea. If the respiratory muscles are the cause of the problem, it is called central sleep apnea. If the problem is caused by a blockage in a person's airway, it is called obstructive sleep apnea.

Some older adults suffer from nocturnal myoclonus, or unusual leg movements. This disorder causes them to wake up either completely or for just a few seconds during the night, because of leg twitching. The cause of this, which can affect one or both legs, is not known. Depending upon the severity of the affliction, either medication or simple leg exercises can bring relief.

If you are having problems sleeping or your sleep pattern has changed dramatically, you should consult your doctor. Fortunately, there are several ways to improve the chances of getting a good night's rest.

Tips For A Good Night's Sleep

1. Establish a regular schedule. When possible, go to sleep and get up at the same time each day. Also, if you develop a regular routine before going to sleep, such as reading, watching the late evening news or taking a hot bath, your body will start to wind down at the same time each night.

2. Get regular exercise. Exercise also will help you get a good night's sleep. Try some moderate physical activity at least four hours before bedtime. Regular exercise reduces tension, promotes relaxation and helps induce a more sound, restful sleep.

3. Get fresh air daily. If you do not get outside often, try stepping outside in the afternoon every day. This will help you adjust your internal sleep clock.

4. Watch what you eat and drink. What you consume can affect your sleep habits. Avoid caffeine late in the day, since caffeine is a stimulant that can prevent you from falling asleep. Also avoid monosodium glutamate, or MSG, a common oriental food seasoning. It, too, is a stimulant. Some experts recommend eating only light meals at the end of the day to avoid sleeplessness that can occur when too much rich food is consumed prior to bedtime.

5. Avoid alcohol and cigarettes. Contrary to popular belief, alcohol and cigarettes do not help you fall asleep. While alcohol is a depressant, research has shown that alcohol disrupts the sleep cycle and robs you of restful sleep. Nicotine in cigarettes is a stimulant that will keep you awake. For safety, always avoid smoking at bedtime.

6. Avoid using your bedroom for anything but sleeping. This helps prevent being distracted before falling asleep. By creating a comfortable environment in your bedroom, you will be able to sleep better. Block out any nonessential noise or light, and make sure you have a telephone close to the bed. A bedside lamp or light switch within easy reach as well as a smoke alarm on each floor of your residence may help you feel more secure, allowing you to get adequate rest.

7. Check your mattress. A comfortable mattress is essential for a good night's sleep. If your mattress is eight to 10 years old, it may need to be replaced. Try putting a sheet of plywood between the mattress and box spring to increase support and make your bed more comfortable.

8. Don't lie in bed wide awake. If you go to bed and find you are still awake after about 15 minutes, get out of bed and do something in another room until you become sleepy. Try putting your mind at ease by clearing your head, thinking relaxing thoughts, listening to some mellow music or reading.

Proper rest is necessary for good health, so don't take sleep for granted. Make sure you take steps to assure a good night's rest every night. If you do all the things listed above and still experience problems sleeping, it may be wise for you to consult your doctor.

CHAPTER NINE

Cover Up In The Sun To Prevent Skin Cancer

Every year more than 500,000 Americans discover they have skin cancer, according to the American Cancer Society. Of that number, more than 27,000 will be diagnosed with malignant melanoma, the deadliest form of skin cancer and a disease that's expected to kill 6,300 people annually.

Doctors discover an increasing number of skin cancer cases each year. This trend is being blamed on the popularity of having tanned skin and the subsequent hours people spend under the sun's harmful rays. Additional blame is being placed on the depletion of the earth's ozone layer. When the ozone layer is depleted from pollution in the atmosphere and other causes, more ultraviolet rays, which damage the skin, reach the earth's surface. According to the Environmental Protection Agency, ozone depletion will cause an additional 4 million cases of skin cancer and 65,000 cancer deaths before the year 2075.

As people get older, they often have more time for leisure and recreational activities, such as golfing, fishing, bicycling or just sitting by the pool. To avoid damaging your skin and to protect against skin cancer, it is extremely important to protect your body from the sun's cancer-causing ultraviolet A and B rays. Ultraviolet rays also can damage your eyes. They need protection from the sun, as well.

Ultraviolet A (UVA) is a long wave version of the sun's radiation which penetrates deeply into the layers of skin, causing tanning, sunburn and aging of the skin. It may be linked to skin cancer. Ultraviolet B (UVB) is a shorter wave of radiation responsible for sunburn, premature aging and wrinkling of the skin, as well as different forms of skin cancer, such as basal-cell, squamous-cell and malignant melanoma.

Basal-cell cancer is considered the most common form of skin cancer and is linked to excessive exposure to the sun. This form of cancer, which develops slowly, is 100-percent curable if diagnosed early and properly treated. Basal-cell cancer rarely spreads and is not likely to form tumors in other parts of the body. While basal-cell carcinomas are rarely fatal, they require attention and treatment by a qualified physician.

Squamous-cell cancer is considered more dangerous, yet is still curable when diagnosed and treated early. This form of cancer develops from keratoses, or small scaly spots which are considered warning signs on skin that has been overexposed to the sun. The keratoses eventually become red or pink warty growths that may be scaly or open in the center and ooze. Squamous-cell cancer can spread and form life-threatening tumors.

The most dangerous form of skin cancer is malignant melanoma. Melanomas are the warning signs for this form of cancer. They are asymmetrical-shaped spots which begin from moles or form on previously unblemished skin. Melanoma spots are light brown or black and may turn partly red, white or blue or become crusty and bleed. Once spots have grown to the size of a dime, the cancer has probably spread to other parts of the body.

Damage to the skin from the sun's rays accumulates over many years and is irreversible. Unfortunately, most people do not realize they have damaged their skin until it is too late, and warning signs start to appear. Malignant melanoma may take 10 to 20 years to appear after the skin has been damaged by the sun.

Ninety percent of all skin cancers occur in areas of the skin that are not covered or protected from the sun. Always consult your doctor if you detect suspicious blemishes on your skin. Skin cancers can be prevented by observing some simple rules and taking precautions to prevent over exposure to UVA and UVB rays.

Stay Out Of The Sun From 10 AM To 3 PM

The most dangerous time of the day to be exposed to sunlight is from 10 a.m. to 3 p.m., when the sun's rays are most intense. If possible, avoid extensive outdoor activity during this time. If you must be in the sun during this time period, there are several ways to protect yourself from the sun's harmful rays.

Proper Clothing

Wear clothing of tightly woven fabric to protect your arms and legs. Long-sleeved, light-weight shirts and long pants or skirts provide the best coverage. Also, wear a hat with a brim or visor and stay in the shade whenever possible. Always remember to cover up in the sun. By doing so, you definitely can reduce your chances of getting skin cancer.

Sunglasses

When it comes to buying a pair of sunglasses to protect your eyes from the sun, cost is not the only factor to consider. Prices for sunglasses range from $4 to $700, or more. Sunglasses are available with colored, mirrored or clear lenses and come in many shapes and sizes. Cost does not necessarily determine effectiveness at blocking out the sun's harmful rays. You can purchase an effective pair of sunglasses for under $10. In choosing a good pair of sunglasses, make sure that the lenses block out at least 75 percent of visible light and block out as much UV radiation as possible. Tinting does affect the amount of visible light that is blocked, however, it does not add protection from UV rays.

There are no set standards for the labeling of sunglasses in the United States. However, some manufacturers do label their products in accordance with the guidelines of the American National Standard Institute (ANSI). When possible, buy sunglasses labeled in one of the following three categories:

General Purpose: Use these in any outdoor activity. Lenses have a dark to medium tint and are suitable for general outdoor use.

Special Purpose: These glasses are designed to protect against bright light. Use them when skiing, mountain climbing or at the beach.

Cosmetic. These glasses feature lightly tinted lenses, and should not be used when exposed to bright sunlight.

Here are some general rules to follow when trying to find an effective pair of sunglasses:

1. When trying on sunglasses, look for lenses dark enough so you cannot see your eyes in the mirror. However, lenses that are too dark can affect or even block your vision.

2. When choosing colored lenses, make sure they do not distort colors to the point that you might not be able to recognize a stop sign or traffic signal.

3. Check the lenses for distortion of shapes, lines and colors. To check if a lens is distorted, hold the glasses at arm's length and look through the lenses at a distant straight line. As you move the glasses across the line, make sure that they don't cause it to bend or sway, indicating a distortion in the lens.

4. Lens and frame size are a matter of preference. Make sure, however, that the frames are large enough to block light on all sides of the frame. Be cautioned against lenses that might effect or impair your peripheral vision, or your ability to see from side to side and top to bottom.

5. If you wear prescription glasses, you may wish to have a pair made for outdoor wear that provides UV-ray protection. Check with your eye doctor or optical store for advice on selecting the best prescription sunglasses for your needs.

Sunscreen

Choosing a sunscreen can be more confusing than finding a pair of sunglasses. Unless you never go outside, there always will be parts of your skin exposed to the sun, especially during leisure activities. When choosing a sunscreen product, look for the Sun Protection Factor (SPF) number. This is a measurement of the amount of UV-ray protection provided by the product. Simply put, the higher the SPF number the longer you can stay safely in the sun without damaging your skin. For example, a sunscreen rated SPF 4 allows you to stay safely in the sun four times longer than you could stay safely with unprotected skin.

There are different points of view on the effectiveness of products with various SPF ratings. SPF numbers range from two to 50. Some experts claim that using a sunscreen with a SPF number of 15 is adequate and using products rated higher is useless and may cause skin irritation. Others say that you should use products with a minimum SPF number of 15 or higher, especially if you have sensitive skin, suffer allergic reactions to the sun or often are exposed to the sun's rays.

For proper protection, apply sunscreen about 45 minutes before going out into the sun. Early application allows the protective chemicals to absorb into the skin. Reapply sunscreen after swimming or profuse sweating. Reapplication also applies to those products that are waterproof, since they may be rubbed off when you use your towel or wipe your brow.

Take steps to protect yourself from the sun's rays at all times. You can get burned even in the shade from rays bouncing off sand or water. Be cautious when it is cloudy outside too, since damaging UV rays can penetrate the cloud cover and burn your skin.

Covering up in the sun helps prevent skin cancer and helps you look your best. Covering up your face helps avoid deep wrinkles and the weathered look that comes from skin damaged by too much exposure to harmful rays of the sun.

CHAPTER TEN

Limit Alcohol / Take Medications Carefully

Alcohol is one of America's most widely used drugs. Surveys indicate that more than two-thirds (66 percent) of adult Americans drink alcohol. As people age, however, surveys show the percentage of adults consuming alcohol declines. Results from a poll conducted for the National Institute on Alcohol Abuse and Alcoholism showed that 45 percent of those surveyed over age 65 consume alcohol.

Many problems are associated with the consumption of alcohol. Drinking alcohol affects both mental and physical health and a person's ability to perform such routine functions as speaking, concentrating, writing and driving. The connection between alcohol and auto accidents has been widely publicized. In the United States, studies show alcohol is a factor in more than 50 percent of all traffic accidents studied.

Individual alcohol consumption levels are measured by Blood Alcohol Content (BAC), which is the percentage of alcohol present in the total blood volume. Body size, age and gender are determining factors. A larger person has more body fluids to dilute the alcohol in the body, which enables that person to drink more without feeling the effects than someone who is smaller. Alcohol has a stronger effect on older adults because seniors have reduced amounts of fluids in their bodies. As a result, it takes much less alcohol to affect an older adult than a younger adult of the same physical size and weight. Men also have more body fluids than women of the same weight, allowing males to consume more without reaching as high a BAC.

Medical research has shown that alcohol impairs normal body functions by affecting the entire central nervous system. According to information contained in the book *Alcohol and Behavior* by Dennison, Prevet and Affleck, one drink of 100-proof alcohol, one 4-ounce glass of wine or one 12-ounce beer, at a BAC of 0.01 to 0.03, causes an average-sized person to feel warm and happy and has a mild-tranquilizing effect. A person who has had two drinks reaches a BAC of 0.05 to 0.06 and becomes more relaxed, begins having trouble with fine motor skills, experiences reduced reaction time and impaired mental performance. After consuming three drinks, BAC reaches 0.08, and a person can experience trouble with vision, hearing, coordination and especially the ability to drive. In some states, driving with a BAC of 0.08 is illegal. A person who is caught driving in this condition is considered legally drunk and can be fined, have his or her driver's license revoked or suspended and may face going to jail. Driving with a BAC of 0.10 is illegal in all states.

Here are a few myths associated with the consumption of alcohol:

Myth: Alcohol is a stimulant. Actually it is a depressant which affects the brain and central nervous system in varying degrees depending on the quantity ingested.

Myth: Alcohol affects everyone in the same way. The effects of alcohol depend on many variables, including the amount and type of alcohol consumed, age, gender and size of the person drinking, whether or not the person has any food in his or her system and whether or not the person has built up a tolerance to alcohol from repeated use.

Myth: Alcohol makes people friendlier. On the contrary, drinking alcohol has been linked to many aggressive behaviors.

Myth: Coffee can "sober up" someone who is intoxicated. The only way someone can "sober up" is through the process of metabolism performed by the liver. The caffeine in coffee is a stimulant which may keep an intoxicated person awake, but it will not affect BAC or the person's ability to function.

Myth: Alcohol is a food supplement. Actually, alcohol does contain a lot of calories, but no vitamins, minerals or protein. The calories in alcohol are used as an energy supply by the body, and as a result other calories obtained from regular foods are not used and are stored as fat. This can lead to weight gain in people who drink heavily on a regular basis. The following chart from the United States Department of Agriculture's Dietary Guidelines for Americans shows the caloric content of some common alcoholic beverages:

BEVERAGE	CALORIES
Beer	
regular, 12 oz.	150
light, 12 oz.	95
Liquor	
gin, rum, vodka	
and whiskey (86-proof), 1 oz. (jigger)	105
vermouth, sweet, 1 oz. (jigger)	70
vermouth, dry, 1 oz. (jigger)	55
Wine, sweet, 5 oz.	200
dry table, white, 5 oz.	115
dry table, red, 5 oz.	110
Cordial and Liqueurs, 1 oz. (jigger)	145

(This chart shows calorie counts for alcoholic drinks only and does not include calories added with mixers.)

If You Do Drink, Do So In Moderation

A moderate amount of alcohol can be consumed without causing any physical or psychological damage. A healthy person usually can have one or two drinks daily without experiencing any long-term health effects. However, when a person becomes a heavy drinker or becomes dependent on alcohol, his or her health, relationships, social functioning and economic status can be affected.

Excessive alcohol consumption has been linked to health problems in all body systems, including the heart, muscles, blood, tissues, brain and digestive track. Alcohol has been associated with the onset of cancer, sexual dysfunction and disrupted sleep patterns. It also suppresses one's desire to eat, which can lead to malnutrition and problems of the liver, kidneys, stomach and heart.

Many older adults often do not eat a proper diet, regardless of alcohol use. A poor diet can be attributed to the inability to cook or to a reduced appetite from a loss of taste due to medication use. As a result, when elderly persons drink excessively, they increase the risk of acquiring nutrition-related illnesses and diseases.

Surveys of the total adult population indicate that the elderly have a smaller percentage of alcoholism when compared to other age groups. However, these surveys may not tell the whole story, since many older adults responding to the survey may not realize they are alcoholics. Also, many health problems associated with excessive alcohol consumption could be masked by existing health problems.

Drug Use And Abuse

In addition to alcohol consumption, older adults also must be cautious about using prescription and non-prescription drugs. Older adults consume the largest percent of all drugs prescribed by physicians. Seniors often have multiple health problems such as arthritis, high blood pressure and heart disease, along with mental problems such as stress, depression and anxiety. In addition, the elderly often are attended to by several different medical specialists, each prescribing medications for one particular health problem. Many of the drug-related health problems seen in older adults stem from interactions, side effects and excessive use of medications prescribed for them by various health care professionals.

Most drug misuse and abuse by older adults is associated with prescribed, legal drugs. Unfortunately, many people believe health problems can be treated only with medicine, prescription and non-prescription drugs. Medicines may not be the best course of action. In fact, many health problems can be solved or relieved with proper diet, exercise, weight loss, counseling and the elimination of smoking and excessive alcohol use. The medical field currently is conducting research to establish the scope of drug abuse among older adults and to develop ways to combat and prevent it.

If you take prescription drugs, keep an accurate record of what you take. By doing so, you will be able to keep your doctors informed of all your medications and avoid any possible side effects or problems caused by mixing prescriptions and over-the-counter drugs. Record the drugs you take in the last section of this handbook.

Also, be aware of the possible side effects of any current medications you take. Carefully follow your doctor's instructions for prescribed drugs. Some drugs should be taken with food, others on an empty stomach. Some cause drowsiness, others cause stomach problems. Always make sure you do not take medication that is outdated. If you have any questions regarding prescription and non-prescription medications, ask your doctor.

Your pharmacist also is a valuable source of information about the medications you take. In fact, pharmacists can alert you to any contraindications of prescription drugs and the effects of taking several different drugs at the same time.

Additionally, avoid mixing alcohol with any form of medication. Taken together, the combination of certain drugs and alcohol could have serious side effects and may be fatal. If you have any questions about the interaction of alcohol and medications you take, ask your doctor or pharmacist.

It is important to be completely informed about any medicine your doctor prescribes for you, keep good records and follow your doctor's orders. When taken properly, prescription and non-prescription drugs are safe and can be beneficial to your health.

CHAPTER ELEVEN

Control Stress

The ability to manage stressful situations in a positive way is critical to maintaining good health. The damaging effects of uncontrolled stress on health have been well documented. Many believe that the accumulation of the effects of stress over a lifetime is a major contributing factor to poor mental and physical health later in life. Stress is so commonplace and routine in our society that many don't recognize when they are under stress.

The assumption that stress is eliminated after a person retires from employment is false. Older adults face many stress-causing situations brought on by such major life disruptions as changes in health, retirement, family living quarters or the loss of a loved one. Learning to handle these situations and to control the stress that is associated with them is the best way to maintain a healthy mental attitude and reduce the chances of damaging your physical health.

Stress is the mental, physical and emotional reactions people have to events or things in their lives that force them to adapt or change. Some suggest that stress is brought on when what you need from life and what you are getting from life are two different things. For example, if you need to work and are recently retired or if you need companionship and are lonely, you may experience stress and anxiety.

Not all stress is bad. Some forms of stress actually may help to motivate people to take on something new or to change in a positive way. Meeting a new friend, learning a new hobby, taking a tour, preparing for a holiday or a visit from a friend can be good sources of stress. Without any stress in our lives, there would be little for which to look forward and to keep us active. However, there are many sources of stress that are not positive, such as the death of a family member or friend, a heated argument, troublesome financial concerns or just a major change in daily routine brought on by retirement, illness or change of living quarters.

The mind and the body are connected. Experiencing too much stress at one time, either good or bad, can cause an accumulation of tension and anxiety that can lead to physical and emotional problems. Hormones which regulate body chemistry are affected by stress and changes in hormone function can cause physical and mental problems. Stress-related health problems frequently include headaches, backaches, muscle tension, fatigue, indigestion, constipation, concentration problems, anger, hostility, eating problems and frustration with even the most minor problems or annoyances. People often experience these symptoms when faced with too much stress.

Some people begin to lose sleep or lose their appetite when confronted with too much stress. Some use alcohol or drugs, while others eat or smoke excessively when feeling stressful. These behaviors rarely eliminate the source of stress and actually may increase it, as well as produce harmful side effects.

A limited amount of stress in our lives properly challenges us and keeps us mentally healthy. However, when stress becomes overwhelming, it's important to know what steps to take to reduce it.

As an older adult, you have a lifetime of experience to draw on in finding ways to cope with stress. Even so, actively seeking ways to limit stress to tolerable levels can help to maintain and even improve your overall health. Here are some suggestions for starting a stress reduction program.

Identify Sources Of Stress

What is stressful to one person may not be stressful to another. Realizing that you are under stress and understanding the cause is the first step toward learning stress management. Identify the sources of stress in your life in order to reduce the stress level. Some common sources of stress and the amounts of stress they cause in most people are listed below. Your reaction to common stress-producing events may be completely different from that of your spouse or neighbor. In addition, there are many other stress producing events, not identified on the list, that may cause stress in your life. Once you have reviewed the chart, list the events or activities that cause you stress. Once they are identified, you can take steps to reduce the impact they have on you.

High Stress Causing Events

Major illness/hospitalization
Death of a loved one
Financial difficulty/Incurring major debt
Divorce
Moving to another state
Problems with the IRS
Legal difficulties
Sex problems
Speaking before a group

Retirement
Marriage
Incurring major debt
Moving

Medium Stress Causing Events

Vacations
A new grandchild
Minor illness
Arguments
Auto repairs/inspections
Dealing with adult children
Holidays

Low Stress Causing Events

Housework
Doctor's appointment
Traffic jams
Poor weather
Meeting new people
Attempting new activities
Going someplace unfamiliar

List Stress Causing Events In Your Life

_____	_____
_____	_____
_____	_____
_____	_____
_____	_____

Control Stress Whenever Possible

Avoid stressful situations whenever possible. However, when you must face stress in your life, try to do so when you feel your best. If you can anticipate stressful periods, you will be able to plan ahead for them. This is not always possible, nevertheless you are better able to handle problems or new situations when you are not tired or feeling ill. Also, when possible, plan for individual events and activities which you feel may be stressful. Think about ways to manage them. Concentrate on the positive aspects, so you will be ready to handle them when they occur.

Problem Solving

Everyone has problems. Learning effective problem-solving skills can dramatically reduce stress. Good problem-solving techniques usually incorporate the following steps. First, identify the crux of the problem by going beyond the surface difficulty or the symptoms to the heart of the matter. Be sure you completely understand the nature of the problem. Then, break the problem into manageable pieces, so each piece can be tackled individually. Gather all the information you need to determine your options and possible solutions. Then, select the best option and go with it. Deal with problems right away, when they are still small.

Set Priorities

Establish priorities so you will know which situation to handle first. Avoid handling too many problems or activities at the same time. Take on commitments you can handle easily and for which you can put forth your best effort. Also, learn to say "no." Do not over commit yourself. Make sure you have enough time to do what is important to you.

One way to take charge of your life is to keep an appointment calendar and set limits on the activities and commitments you schedule.

Look For Support

Talking with others can help clear confusion and eliminate fear that often comes with change. If you need help with a problem or just have something that's on your mind, talk to a family member or a friend. Don't be afraid to ask for help when you need it. But remember, good relationships are two-way streets. Get back in touch with good friends and family members that have drifted away and try to patch up troubled relationships. Giving help is as important as receiving it. If you share your feelings, you may find others who have faced similar problems. They probably will have some good advice for you on how to handle the stress. Many people also have found support in their religious beliefs.

Exercise!

Exercise is one of the best ways to get rid of stress. If done regularly, exercise decreases anxiety and depression. Take a walk, go for a swim, ride a bike, go dancing. Find something that helps keep both your body and your mind healthy and active.

Learn To Relax!

Here's an exercise that will help you "wind down" when you are "stressed out." Lie down or sit in a comfortable chair. Close your eyes and take slow, deep breaths. Begin at your toes and tighten the muscles. Hold them tight for a moment. Then as you relax the muscles, let go of the tension. Do the same thing with the rest of your body, progressively moving up from your toes to your head. When your entire body is relaxed, rest quietly.

If you feel overwhelmed, take a break and do something fun. Read a book, see a movie, take a vacation or just go out of town for a few days. If you can't physically leave town, try a good daydream. Close your eyes and transplant yourself to somewhere relaxing or enjoyable. Imagine all the sights, sounds, people, smells and activities that are part of the place in your daydream. Relax for a while, and live in your thoughts. A mini-massage of the neck, shoulders and head also helpes to relax and relieve stressful tension.

Eat Right

Stress can burn extra calories and weaken your immune system. Getting enough of the recommended nutrients in your body is always important, but it is essential during times of stress. Eating right will keep up your energy level and better prepare you to face a stressful situation. Some people overeat when feeling stressed. Overeating can lead to obesity, which is linked directly to many serious health problems. If you overeat when you feel stressed, try relaxation techniques or exercise instead of eating.

Get Plenty Of Rest

If stress is keeping you awake, try adjusting your bedtime routine and avoid caffeine late in the day. Try to complete tasks before you going to bed so an unfinished task won't bother you and keep you awake. Avoid strenuous activity close to bedtime. Start winding down and relaxing about 30 minutes before you plan to go to sleep.

A good sleeping environment contributes to sound sleep and proper rest. Make sure the room temperature, lighting and bed surface are just right for you. If music relaxes you, choose some that will help you wind down. Also, try drinking some warm milk or herb tea.

Keep Control of Your Life

You can be independent even as you grow older. Aging doesn't mean illness and dependence necessarily. Make time for yourself and use the time to plan for changes that will make your life less stressful. When you face major decisions, find out all the facts and don't make hasty decisions or accept unnecessary limitations. Do what feels right for you! The more control you maintain over your life, the less stressful it will be.

These tips can help you cope with daily stress causing situations. However, events may occur which normal stress management techniques cannot handle effectively. It's perfectly normal to be very upset about the loss of a loved one or after facing a major crisis or change. Some people take longer to recover from major stress causing events than others. If stress-related symptoms continue for more than a few months, or if you are experiencing frequent crying spells, feelings of hopelessness, loss of control over your life or thoughts of suicide, seek professional help. It takes time to recover from certain challenges in life and some may require additional professional support and guidance.

CHAPTER TWELVE

Be Positive/ Enjoy People

A positive mental attitude is a key factor in healthy aging. Adults who understand and cope with the process of getting older - adjusting to retirement, losing some physical ability and adapting to major life changes - are better able to physically and mentally handle the challenges they may face. Older adults who maintain a positive mental attitude about living continue to profit from interactions with others, remain active, set new goals and find life meaningful.

Scientists have established a link between physical and mental health. They have found a person's mental attitude or disposition is a major factor in how disease and illness affect an individual. Studies of people suffering from a severe or chronic illness have often shown a significant difference between the progress of those with a positive mental attitude and the progress of those with a negative one. With all other factors being relatively equal, people maintaining positive mental attitudes were found to be in better physical and mental health than those who were not positive. An old saying reminds us that people who have a positive outlook on life and remain active haven't time to get sick or dwell on their infirmities.

Stereotypes about older adults cover all aspects of daily living and make it difficult for older individuals to separate themselves from the generalizations about how seniors are supposed to act and live their lives. These generalizations sometimes depict seniors as fragile, weak, dependent, poverty-stricken and unhappy. Another generalization suggests that older adults must socialize constantly and always be with others to be happy. It is not easy for many older adults to establish their own identity and divorce themselves from such stereotypes and generalizations. Having a positive attitude about aging helps avoid falling into the stereotypical behavior often associated with seniors.

According to reports by specialists in the field, there are five components of life's satisfaction for older adults:

1. The individual takes pleasure from whatever activities constitute his or her everyday life -- that is, the person who enjoys sitting at home and watching television can be as satisfied as the person who starts a second career or new business venture after retiring.

2. The individual regards his or her life as meaningful and accepts responsibility for what life has been and continues to be.

3. The person feels that he or she has succeeded in achieving major goals in life.

4. The individual holds a positive self-image as a worthwhile person, regardless of present physical condition.

5. The individual maintains optimistic attitudes and moods.

Recent studies indicate older adults maintain many of the same tendencies and attitudes held during their entire lives. Many, however develop new ideals and attitudes once they are freed from the required obligations or expectations of a career and/or societal standing. New attitudes and ideals often lead to new interests and activities that can be stimulating and rewarding. Seniors should recognize that once they turn 65, they do not automatically have to assume the role of the "nice old man" or the "sweet old lady" whose only ambitions are to feed the pigeons in the park or to play cards all day, unless that is what they choose to do.

Maintaining a positive mental attitude, high self-esteem and the ability to communicate with others is essential to healthy aging. Good mental health also requires acceptance by an individual of his or her capabilities and limitations. There are many ways for people to change their attitude and be more positive. The following suggestions may be helpful in developing a positive outlook.

Set New Goals

Having goals to achieve and obligations to fulfill give meaning and purpose to everyone's life. Few older people are completely satisfied with their life's accomplishments and most will admit they probably fell short of fulfilling some of their major life goals. For example, a person with a successful career may not have reached the very top of his or her profession, or a parent who has successfully raised a family may not be entirely happy with how the children turned out as adults. Older adults should not feel because they have reached retirement or have raised their families they have nothing else to accomplish. What is really important and meaningful is the process of working toward a goal, not just reaching it.

Setting goals and objectives forces people to focus attention on things they want to accomplish. Human energy and effort are directed to the positive activities necessary to achieve them. New life goals can be established at any age. For example, goals might include such diverse things as visiting all 50 states of the United States, learning to play a musical instrument, writing the family history, learning to use a computer, or volunteering time to a group or organization. The important thing is making a commitment and taking pleasure in working toward a goal.

See Change As Opportunity

All seniors face many major changes in their lives as they age. These include retirement, moving to new living quarters, children growing up and leaving home and some diminished physical abilities. Look at each event as a new opportunity to experience life. People who are open to change often find their lives enriched by new experiences and acquaintances encountered as a result of a change. By looking for opportunities in change, you are helping to develop a positive attitude.

Enjoy Other People

Good communication skills and the ability to socialize with others help maintain self-esteem and make it easier to enjoy others. Other people can contribute to a person's positive outlook. Interacting with people of all ages gives seniors a chance to exchange experience, knowledge and expertise.

People of any age naturally seek companionship and have a need to feel the love and touch of others. Companionship is necessary for giving and receiving support. A positive attitude can be strengthened if one seeks the company of other positive people.

The very elderly often find themselves more and more dependent on others for transportation, personal care, a place to live and meals. This dependence can be hard to accept for those who have been independent most of their lives. Developing a good relationship with caregivers and learning to enjoy their company, as well as accept their assistance, can help to cultivate a positive attitude.

Spend Quality Time Alone

People can experience happiness, pleasure and personal fulfillment without the constant presence of others. Adequate privacy is necessary for maintaining mental abilities that are required to cope with others and to accomplish personal goals and tasks that require concentration. The amount of time spent alone necessary to reinforce a positive mental attitude varies among individuals. Determine how much time you need to spend alone and plan for this time in your daily or weekly schedule.

Seek Spiritual Comfort

As people grow older, their perception of life and its events may change. Some will begin to view life in a more spiritual way and look to either formal or informal religion to help understand and cope with later years. A spiritual outlook has given meaning and purpose to many and can have a very positive impact on a person's physical and mental condition. Spiritualism can bring peace of mind, especially to those with few family members, friends and associates to confide in.

A good outlook on life may be the single most important factor in helping to maintain good physical and mental health. Enormous benefits can be derived from a positive mental attitude and a sincere enjoyment of other people.

CHAPTER THIRTEEN

Get Regular Check-ups

Many healthcare professionals are changing their opinions about the annual physical exam and other health check-ups. Most no longer recommend that everyone have a complete exam every year. Younger healthy adults may need a thorough, routine physical exam only every few years, along with periodic health evaluations. Healthy, older adults, however, should get a physical exam every year. The exam will include several screening examinations and tests.

Screening examinations and tests are performed to provide early detection of disease or other health problems. As people age, their chances of developing health problems increase. Screening tests and evaluation procedures often can detect health problems, even before a person experiences any noticeable symptoms. Generally speaking, doctors usually recommend that older adults have screening tests and procedures done more frequently because they are at greater risk for developing certain diseases or conditions.

Some tests, such as an electrocardiogram or a chest x-ray, are done to provide physicians and other healthcare professionals with baseline information with which to compare later tests. Other tests, such as those for blood pressure, blood count, urinalysis and cholesterol level, are done to give healthcare professionals information about the patient's current state of health.

If a patient has a health risk, a doctor may recommend certain tests or screening examinations be done more frequently than advised for the average, healthy person. For example, if a patient has a health problem that could lead to a more serious complication, a doctor may advise that tests for the problem be conducted frequently. Likewise, if there is a family history of certain diseases or health problems, a doctor probably will advise evaluations be done more often than normally recommended.

Remember, the purpose of health screening tests and examinations is to assist in early detection of health problems. Early diagnosis and treatment are important for the successful medical management of health problems.

Self Examination

In addition to examinations and screening tests conducted by a healthcare professional, you can do several things to check your health by yourself. Women should do a breast self-examination every month. Men should perform testicular self-exams. If you are not familiar with these exams, ask your doctor to show you how to perform them.

Frequently check your skin when showering or bathing for any changes in warts or moles or any blemishes that could signal the onset of skin cancer. Routinely examine your mouth, teeth and gums when brushing your teeth.

People who take charge of their health and get periodic health check-ups can increase their chances for long and healthy lives.

Suggested Health Screening Procedures
For Healthy Females Over 60 Years of Age

Suggested Test	Examination Frequency	My Doctors Recommend
History & Physical	Yearly	_____
Height & Weight	Yearly	_____
Eye Exam	Yearly	_____
Dental Exam	Yearly	_____
Hearing Test	Every 5 Years	_____
Urinalysis	Every 2 Years	_____
Blood Count	Every 2 years	_____
Blood Sugar	Yearly	_____
Cholesterol Level	Once for baseline	_____
Rectal Exam	Yearly	_____
Colon Exam	Yearly	_____
Stool Test for Blood	Yearly	_____
Thyroid Test	Every 2 years	_____
Electrocardiogram	Once for baseline	_____
Chest x-ray	Once for baseline	_____
Breast Self-Exam	Monthly	_____
Breast Exam -Physician	Yearly	_____
Mammogram	Yearly	_____
Pelvic Exam	Yearly	_____
Pap Smear	Yearly	_____
Blood Pressure	Yearly	_____

Suggested Health Screening Procedures
For Healthy Males Over 60 Years of Age

Suggested Test	Examination Frequency	My Doctors Recommend
History & Physical	Yearly	_____
Height & Weight	Yearly	_____
Eye Exam	Yearly	_____
Dental Exam	Yearly	_____
Hearing Test	Every 5 Years	_____
Urinalysis	Every 2 Years	_____
Blood Count	Every 2 years	_____
Blood Sugar	Yearly	_____
Cholesterol Level	Once for baseline	_____
Rectal Exam	Yearly	_____
Colon Exam	Yearly	_____
Stool Test for Blood	Yearly	_____
Thyroid Test	Every 2 years	_____
Electrocardiogram	Once for baseline	_____
Chest x-ray	Once for baseline	_____
Blood Pressure	Yearly	_____
Prostrate Exam	Yearly	_____
Testicular Self-Exam	Monthly	_____
Testicular Exam -Physician	Yearly	_____

CHAPTER FOURTEEN

Keeping Accurate Medical Records

Keeping accurate medical records can help you manage your medical care and assist healthcare professionals in monitoring your health status. Don't rely on your memory alone to keep track of all the information that relates to your health.

Use this handbook to write down important information. List the health professionals you have seen and why, illnesses or surgeries you have had, medications you have taken, instructions from your doctors or other health care professionals and the results of screening tests and examinations.

Take this handbook with you whenever you visit your doctor. Carefully record your doctor's instructions so you can follow them exactly. If your doctor's office routinely takes your blood pressure and checks your weight, record the results in this handbook with every visit. Also, store important medical records in the pocket envelope provided in this section. Refer to the handbook, if necessary, to answer your doctor's questions about your health. This is especially important if you are seeing a new physician or health-care provider that is not familiar with your medical background and history.

Keep the book in a safe place and let someone know its whereabouts in case of a medical emergency.

Take this handbook with you when you travel. In case of a medical emergency, you or your traveling companions can use the information in the book to quickly supply medical professionals with accurate information that can assist with your treatment.

Finally, keep pertinent or current medical insurance information handy for easy reference in the pockets provided. Since healthcare is costly, you should review your coverage to make sure you know exactly what your insurance plan(s) covers.

Health Care Professionals

Keep a list of your doctors and other health care providers here.

DOCTORS

Speciality:_____

Name:_____

Address:_____

City: _____State:_____Zip:_____

Phone:_____

Speciality:_____

Name:_____

Address:_____

City: _____State:_____Zip:_____

Phone:_____

Speciality:_____

Name:_____

Address:_____

City: _____State:_____Zip:_____

Phone:_____

Speciality:_____

Name:_____

Address:_____

City: _____State:_____Zip:_____

Phone:_____

Speciality:_____

Name:_____

Address:_____

City: _____State:_____Zip:_____

Phone:_____

Speciality:_____

Name:_____

Address:_____

City: _____State:_____Zip:_____

Phone:_____

Speciality:_____

Name:_____

Address:_____

City: _____State:_____Zip:_____

Phone:_____

DENTISTS

Name:_____

Address:_____

City: _____State:_____Zip:_____

Phone:_____

Name:_____

Address:_____

City: _____State:_____Zip:_____

Phone:_____

OPTOMETRIST

Name:_____

Address:_____

City: _____State:_____Zip:_____

Phone:_____

OPTICAL STORE

Name:_____

Location:_____

Phone:_____

THERAPISTS

Name:_____

Address:_____

City: _____State:_____Zip:_____

Phone:_____

Name:_____

Address:_____

City: _____State:_____Zip:_____

Phone:_____

Name:_____

Address:_____

City: _____State:_____Zip:_____

Phone:_____

PHARMACY

Name:_____

Location:_____Phone:_____

Name:_____

Location:_____Phone:_____

Record Of Illness & Surgery

Type Of Illness/ Surgery	Date	Hospital/Doctor

Record Of Illness & Surgery

Type Of Illness/ Surgery	Date	Hospital/Doctor

Record Of Illness & Surgery

Type Of Illness/ Surgery	Date	Hospital/Doctor

Record Of Illness & Surgery

Type Of Illness/ Surgery	Date	Hospital/Doctor

Healthcare Provider Visits

Use this section of the handbook to keep track of your visits to healthcare providers and to record instructions and advice given to you by your physician and other healthcare professionals.

*Date:*_____*Visit To:* _____

*Reason For The Visit:*_____

_____

Advice/Instructions: _____

_____

_____

_____

_____

Next Appointment: _____

*Comments To Tell The Doctor at the Next Visit:*_____

_____

_____

_____

_____

_____

*Date:*_____*Visit To:*_____

*Reason For The Visit:*_____

_____

*Advice/Instructions:*_____

_____

_____

_____

_____

_____

*Next Appointment:*_____

*Comments To Tell The Doctor at the Next Visit:*_____

_____

_____

_____

_____

_____

Date:_____Visit To: _____

Reason For The Visit:_____

_____

Advice/Instructions: _____

_____

_____

_____

_____

_____

Next Appointment: _____

Comments To Tell The Doctor at the Next Visit:_____

_____

_____

_____

_____

_____

_____

Date: _____ *Visit To:* _____

Reason For The Visit: _____

_____

Advice/Instructions: _____

_____

_____

_____

_____

_____

Next Appointment: _____

Comments To Tell The Doctor at the Next Visit: _____

_____

_____

_____

_____

_____

_____

Date:_____Visit To: _____

Reason For The Visit:_____

_____

Advice/Instructions: _____

_____

_____

_____

_____

_____

_____

Next Appointment: _____

Comments To Tell The Doctor at the Next Visit:_____

_____

_____

_____

_____

_____

_____

_____

*Date:*_____*Visit To:* _____

*Reason For The Visit:*_____

_____

Advice/Instructions: _____

_____

_____

_____

_____

_____

_____

Next Appointment: _____

*Comments To Tell The Doctor at the Next Visit:*_____

_____

_____

_____

_____

_____

_____

Date:_____Visit To: _____ _____

Reason For The Visit:_____

_____

Advice/Instructions: _____

_____

_____

_____

_____

_____

Next Appointment: _____

Comments To Tell The Doctor at the Next Visit:_____

_____

_____

_____

_____

_____

_____

Date: _____ *Visit To:* _____

Reason For The Visit: _____

_____

Advice/Instructions: _____

_____

_____

_____

_____

_____

_____

Next Appointment: _____

Comments To Tell The Doctor at the Next Visit: _____

_____

_____

_____

_____

_____

_____

_____

*Date:*_____*Visit To:* _____

*Reason For The Visit:*_____

_____

Advice/Instructions: _____

_____

_____

_____

_____

_____

_____

Next Appointment: _____

*Comments To Tell The Doctor at the Next Visit:*_____

_____

_____

_____

_____

_____

_____

*Date:*_____*Visit To:*_____

*Reason For The Visit:*_____

_____

*Advice/Instructions:*_____

_____

_____

_____

_____

_____

_____

*Next Appointment:*_____

*Comments To Tell The Doctor at the Next Visit:*_____

_____

_____

_____

_____

_____

_____

_____

*Date:*_____*Visit To:*_____

*Reason For The Visit:*_____

_____

*Advice/Instructions:*_____

_____

_____

_____

_____

_____

*Next Appointment:*_____

*Comments To Tell The Doctor at the Next Visit:*_____

_____

_____

_____

_____

_____

_____

*Date:*_____*Visit To:* _____

*Reason For The Visit:*_____

_____

Advice/Instructions: _____

_____

_____

_____

_____

_____

_____

Next Appointment: _____

*Comments To Tell The Doctor at the Next Visit:*_____

_____

_____

_____

_____

_____

_____

*Date:*_____*Visit To:* _____

*Reason For The Visit:*_____

_____

Advice/Instructions: _____

_____

_____

_____

_____

_____

_____

Next Appointment: _____

*Comments To Tell The Doctor at the Next Visit:*_____

_____

_____

_____

_____

_____

_____

_____

*Date:*_____*Visit To:*_____

*Reason For The Visit:*_____

_____

*Advice/Instructions:*_____

_____

_____

_____

_____

_____

_____

*Next Appointment:*_____

*Comments To Tell The Doctor at the Next Visit:*_____

_____

_____

_____

_____

_____

_____

Date:_____Visit To: _____

Reason For The Visit:_____

_____

Advice/Instructions: _____

_____

_____

_____

_____

_____

_____

Next Appointment: _____

Comments To Tell The Doctor at the Next Visit:_____

_____

_____

_____

_____

_____

_____

*Date:*_____*Visit To:* _____

*Reason For The Visit:*_____

_____

Advice/Instructions: _____

_____

_____

_____

_____

_____

_____

Next Appointment: _____

*Comments To Tell The Doctor at the Next Visit:*_____

_____

_____

_____

_____

_____

_____

_____

Date:_____Visit To: _____

Reason For The Visit:_____

_____

Advice/Instructions: _____

_____

_____

_____

_____

_____

_____

Next Appointment: _____

Comments To Tell The Doctor at the Next Visit:_____

_____

_____

_____

_____

_____

_____

_____

*Date:*_____*Visit To:* _____

*Reason For The Visit:*_____

_____

Advice/Instructions: _____

_____

_____

_____

_____

_____

Next Appointment: _____

*Comments To Tell The Doctor at the Next Visit:*_____

_____

_____

_____

_____

_____

_____

_____

*Date:*_____*Visit To:* _____

*Reason For The Visit:*_____

_____

Advice/Instructions: _____

_____

_____

_____

_____

_____

Next Appointment: _____

*Comments To Tell The Doctor at the Next Visit:*_____

_____

_____

_____

_____

_____

_____

_____

*Date:*_____*Visit To:* _____

*Reason For The Visit:*_____

_____

Advice/Instructions: _____

_____

_____

_____

_____

_____

Next Appointment: _____

*Comments To Tell The Doctor at the Next Visit:*_____

_____

_____

_____

_____

_____

_____

_____

Date:_____Visit To: _____

Reason For The Visit:_____

_____

Advice/Instructions: _____

_____

_____

_____

_____

_____

Next Appointment: _____

Comments To Tell The Doctor at the Next Visit:_____

_____

_____

_____

_____

_____

_____

Date:_____Visit To: _____

Reason For The Visit:_____

_____

Advice/Instructions: _____

_____

_____

_____

_____

_____

_____

Next Appointment: _____

Comments To Tell The Doctor at the Next Visit:_____

_____

_____

_____

_____

_____

_____

_____

*Date:*_____*Visit To:* _____

*Reason For The Visit:*_____

_____

Advice/Instructions: _____

_____

_____

_____

_____

_____

_____

Next Appointment: _____

*Comments To Tell The Doctor at the Next Visit:*_____

_____

_____

_____

_____

_____

_____

_____

Date:_____Visit To: _____

Reason For The Visit:_____

_____

Advice/Instructions: _____

_____

_____

_____

_____

_____

_____

Next Appointment: _____

Comments To Tell The Doctor at the Next Visit:_____

_____

_____

_____

_____

_____

_____

_____

*Date:*_____*Visit To:*_____

*Reason For The Visit:*_____

_____

*Advice/Instructions:*_____

_____

_____

_____

_____

_____

_____

*Next Appointment:*_____

*Comments To Tell The Doctor at the Next Visit:*_____

_____

_____

_____

_____

_____

_____

_____

Date:_____Visit To: _____

Reason For The Visit:_____

_____

Advice/Instructions: _____

_____

_____

_____

_____

_____

_____

Next Appointment: _____

Comments To Tell The Doctor at the Next Visit:_____

_____

_____

_____

_____

_____

_____

_____

*Date:*_____*Visit To:* _____

*Reason For The Visit:*_____

_____

Advice/Instructions: _____

_____

_____

_____

_____

_____

_____

Next Appointment: _____

*Comments To Tell The Doctor at the Next Visit:*_____

_____

_____

_____

_____

_____

_____

*Date:*_____*Visit To:* _____

*Reason For The Visit:*_____

_____

Advice/Instructions: _____

_____

_____

_____

_____

_____

Next Appointment: _____

*Comments To Tell The Doctor at the Next Visit:*_____

_____

_____

_____

_____

_____

_____

Date:_____Visit To: _____

Reason For The Visit:_____

_____

Advice/Instructions: _____

_____

_____

_____

_____

_____

_____

Next Appointment: _____

Comments To Tell The Doctor at the Next Visit:_____

_____

_____

_____

_____

_____

_____

*Date:*_____*Visit To:* _____

*Reason For The Visit:*_____

_____

Advice/Instructions: _____

_____

_____

_____

_____

_____

Next Appointment: _____

*Comments To Tell The Doctor at the Next Visit:*_____

_____

_____

_____

_____

_____

_____

Medication Record

List all medications you take, along with any special instructions or restrictions. This information is important to you, your family and your doctors. Inform your doctors of all drugs you take.

Date Prescribed	Name of Medicine (generic/brand)	Reason Taken	Dose	How Often	Special Instructions

Medication Record

List all medications you take, along with any special instructions or restrictions. This information is important to you, your family and your doctors. Inform your doctors of all drugs you take.

Date Prescribed	Name of Medicine (generic/brand)	Reason Taken	Dose	How Often	Special Instructions

Medication Record

List all medications you take, along with any special instructions or restrictions. This information is important to you, your family and your doctors. Inform your doctors of all drugs you take.

Date Prescribed	Name of Medicine (generic/brand)	Reason Taken	Dose	How Often	Special Instructions

Medication Record

List all medications you take, along with any special instructions or restrictions. This information is important to you, your family and your doctors. Inform your doctors of all drugs you take.

Date Prescribed	Name of Medicine (generic/brand)	Reason Taken	Dose	How Often	Special Instructions

Medication Record

List all medications you take, along with any special instructions or restrictions. This information is important to you, your family and your doctors. Inform your doctors of all drugs you take.

Date Prescribed	Name of Medicine (generic/brand)	Reason Taken	Dose	How Often	Special Instructions

Medication Record

List all medications you take, along with any special instructions or restrictions. This information is important to you, your family and your doctors. Inform your doctors of all drugs you take.

Date Prescribed	Name of Medicine (generic/brand)	Reason Taken	Dose	How Often	Special Instructions

Health Aids

Eyeglass Prescription:

_____ _____

_____

_____

Hearing Aid:

_____

_____

_____

Dentures:

_____

_____

Other Important Information:

_____

_____

_____

_____

_____

_____

Allergies

List any allergies you have below:

_____

_____

_____

_____

Special Dietary Requirements

List any special dietary requirements or restrictions you have below:

_____

_____

_____

_____

Height Record

Date	Measure	Date	Measure
_____	_____	_____	_____
_____	_____	_____	_____

Immunization Record

Check with your doctor about when to receive immunizations recommended for older adults. These might include a tetanus shot every 10 years, influenza vaccine yearly and pneumonia vaccine. Keep a record of your immunizations here.

Immunization	Dose	Date

Cholesterol Level Record

A cholesterol level below 200 mg/dl is recommended to lower the risk of heart disease.

Date	Cholesterol Count	Location of Test

Cholesterol Level Record

A cholesterol level below 200 mg/dl is recommended to lower the risk of heart disease.

Date	Cholesterol Count	Location of Test

Blood Pressure Readings

Date	Reading	Location of Reading

Blood Pressure Readings

Date	Reading	Location of Reading

Health Insurance Information

List your health insurance policies here for handy reference. Make a duplicate copy of this information to keep in a safe place.

Medical Insurance

Policy Number:_____

Company/Agent:_____

Telephone:_____

Policy Number:_____

Company/Agent:_____

Telephone:_____

Policy Number:_____

Company/Agent:_____

Telephone:_____

Dental Insurance

Policy Number:_____

Company/Agent:_____

Telephone:_____

Optical Insurance

Policy Number:_____

Company/Agent:_____

Telephone:_____

Long Term Care Insurance

Policy Number:_____

Company/Agent:_____

Telephone:_____

Life Insurance & Other

Policy Number:_____

Company/Agent:_____

Telephone:_____

Policy Number:_____

Company/Agent:_____

Telephone:_____

Makes A Great Gift For Friends Or Relatives.

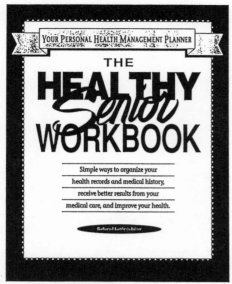

THE HEALTHY SENIOR WORKBOOK is the perfect gift for all occassions. **Extra copies are available at your local bookstore.** Or, you can have a gift copy sent to your favorite seniors along with a gift card simply by completing the order form below.

Mail Order $14.50
(Includes shipping & handling)

[ ] YES! Send a copy of *The Healthy Senior Workbook* to those listed below. Enclosed is a check for $14.50 for each copy or I authorize the use of my credit card.

Gift From:_____ Address:_____

City:_____State:_____ Zip:_____ Telephone:_____

Send To:

Name:_____   Name:_____

Address:_____   Address:_____

City:_____ State:____Zip:_____   City:_____ State:_____ Zip:_____

[ ] Check Enclosed   [ ] MasterCard   [ ] VISA   Amount: $_____

Card #_____   Expiration Date:_____

Signature:_____

Send your order to: **Marketing Methods Press**
1413 E. Marshall Avenue
Phoenix, AZ 85014